TQ

The Art and Science of
Spa & Body
Therapy

WRITTEN BY JANE FOULSTON, ELAINE HALL, FAE MAJOR & MARGUERITE WYNNE

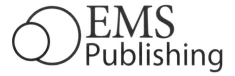

EMS
Publishing

Introduction

The Art and Science of Spa & Body Therapy has been produced with the student in mind. It is clearly written, explaining complex subjects concisely but comprehensively with images and illustrations throughout; it is structured to support the learner in their studies.

The Art and Science of spa & Body Therapy has been written to meet the National Occupational Standards in the UK at Level 3 for spa and body electrical treatments. These standards are reflected in the syllabuses of all the main examination boards that award spa qualifications - BTEC, CIBTAC, CIDESCO, City & Guilds, ITEC & VTCT.

Published by EMS Publishing
2nd Floor Chiswick Gate,
598-608 Chiswick High Road, London, W4 5RT
0845 017 9022

© Education and Media Services Ltd.

First published May 2011

Designed for the publishers by Idego Media Limited
Book, brochure, catalogue and magazine design specialists for print and digital.
More information can be found at www.idegomedia.co.uk

Additional images courtesy of istockphoto.com and alamy.com

Printed by Scot print

ISBN 9781903348123

Acknowledgements

Editor
Jane Foulston

Jane Foulston, the Chief Executive of ITEC, has been working in the in the beauty industry for over 28 years and has edited many best selling textbooks. Jane has always had a passion for education and the need to provide the highest standards of education in the beauty and spa industry.

Sub-Editors
Fae Major

Fae Major has worked in the beauty therapy industry for 23 years. Her experience has included working for Steiner's alternative medicine clinics as well as private beauty salons in the UK and Barbados. Fae has fifteen years' teaching experience and as a result became a practical examiner for ITEC in 1992. As well as continuing to examine, Fae is currently working for ITEC as part of the Qualifications Development team.

Marguerite Wynne

Marguerite Wynne began her career in one of London's foremost beauty salons and went onto teach in the College of Beauty Therapy in London. Subsequently she owned her own salon and school in Buckinghamshire and at the same time worked as Chief Examiner for ITEC. In 2005 Marguerite was appointed Education Manager for ITEC where she now monitors the standards and consistency of ITEC examinations.

Elaine Hall

Elaine Hall began her career teaching beauty and complementary therapies at the West of England College in Bath. She then went on to manage the complementary therapies section at Bridgwater College. Since then Elaine has run her own private salon and clinic based within a nursing home where she has treated both the elderly and private clients. In addition she has held the post of Senior ITEC Examiner and she examines extensively both in the South West of England and overseas, and is part of the qualifications development team.

Also with thanks to:

Carlton Professional and especially to Angela Barbagelata for, help with supplying electrical equipment vital production of this textbook.
For over 60 years The Carlton Group has placed caring for our customers at the heart of our business. Via the Carlton Professional portfolio of products, The Carlton Group offers the security of quality British made electrotherapy machines, furniture and accessories for the beauty and spa industries. For further information call The Carlton Group on 01903 761100 or visit www.thecarltongroup.co.uk

Dove Spa for supplying their fantastic products used throughout this textbook.

Nirvana Spa for their kind permission to use images of their spa facilities.

ES Media for their help with the production of the electronic media.

Copy writing Company for their help with the producing the final text.

Models: Karolina Palasinski, Rachael Kammerling & Sheetal Bhatt

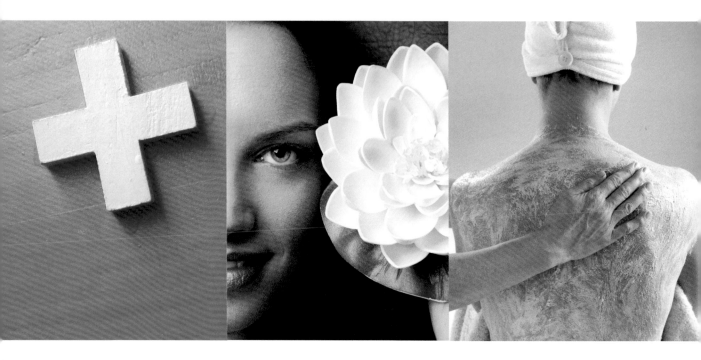

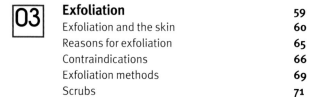

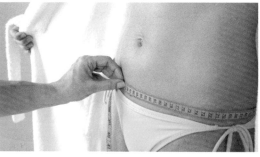

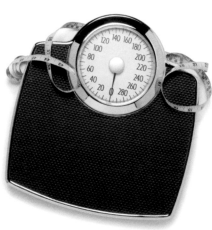

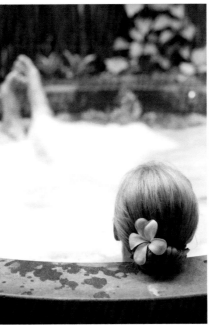

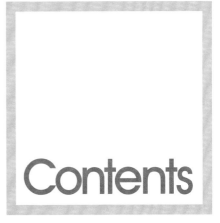

Contents

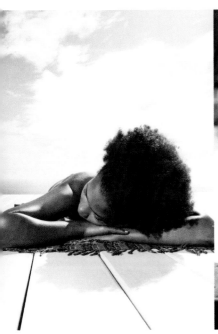

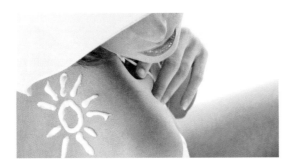

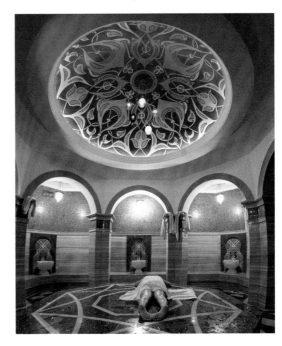

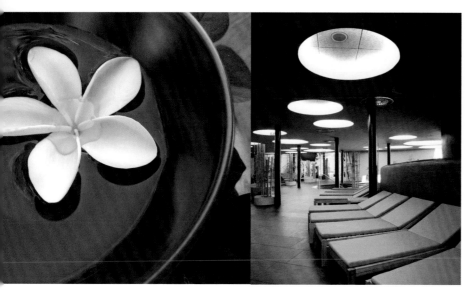

Contents

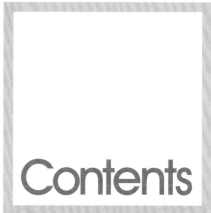

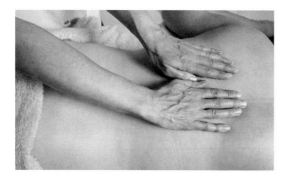

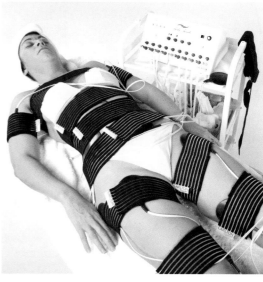

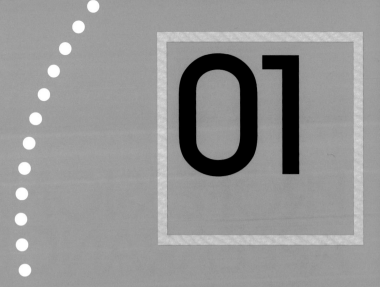

01

Being professional

As a therapist you represent both your profession and your employer and, when clients consult you, they are placing their confidence in you as a professional. They are entrusting their health and wellbeing to your care, and they expect every aspect of the service you provide to be professional. Being professional is about making sure that everything – including your personal presentation, communication and behaviour; the environment in which you work; client care; health and safety and, of course, the treatments you provide – all meet the highest professional standards.

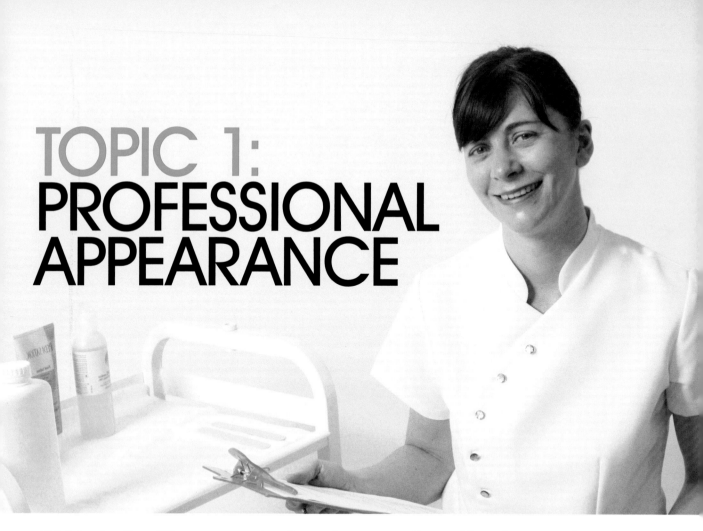

TOPIC 1:
PROFESSIONAL APPEARANCE

Within the first fifteen seconds of meeting, your client will make a number of judgements about you and your abilities, all of which will be based on your attitude and your appearance. For example, if you look untidy and dishevelled a new client may make the assumption that the service you will provide to them is going to be slapdash and careless. However, if you look neat and well groomed, a new client is much more likely to assume that your treatments will be competent and professional.

PERSONAL PRESENTATION

To ensure that you look professional throughout your working day you need to pay careful attention to the following:

1) Personal hygiene

Personal hygiene is a key element of professional presentation. Use a deodorant or anti-perspirant to prevent body odour. Always check that your breath is fresh and sweet smelling on a regular basis. Also ensure that your hair is clean and tied back off the collar and face and that your nails are short, clean and without nail polish.

2) Uniform

A clean and freshly ironed uniform is essential to presenting a professional appearance. If you are working in a salon you will be expected to wear professional work wear. If wearing white at work you will almost certainly need at least three uniforms; one to wear, one to wash and one to keep at work as a spare just in case you have an accident. Nothing looks more untidy or unprofessional than a white uniform that is marked with splashes or stains. It's worth noting that, for reasons of hygiene, many employers will expect you to wear tights or stockings, even during the hot

• KEY POINT

Your appearance should confirm to your clients that you are a professional and qualified therapist and should give them the confidence to enable them to relax, knowing that they are safe in your hands.

summer months. If you wear tights, do make sure that they are plain and a natural colour.

If you are working as a sports therapist, the usual uniform is a polo shirt and tracksuit bottoms. If you are wearing trousers you should choose full, flat shoes and socks of the same colour. It is important always to make sure that you look neat and well groomed.

3) Hair
Hair must be clean and tied back from your face so that it doesn't flop forward or rest on your collar. Tied-back hair will be cooler and more comfortable for you, and will also be more hygienic for the client.

4) Nails and hands
Nails and hands must be kept scrupulously clean. Nails should be neatly trimmed and unvarnished, unless you are a nail technician, in which case your own nails should be regarded as a valuable advertisement for your skills, and maintained accordingly.

5) Make-up
Make-up must be worn and should always look fresh and professionally applied.

6) Perfume
Heavy perfume should be avoided as some clients may find strong odours unpleasant, or may even be allergic to certain fragrances.

7) Shoes
Shoes should be practical and, above all, comfortable as you will be wearing them throughout the working day. Your shoes should have closed toes and heels, and must be flat. As you are likely to be on your feet for long hours it's a good idea to ensure that you have a suitable spare pair that you can change into halfway through the day. This will help to keep your feet fresh and comfortable. It's also a good idea to have spare socks or tights to hand so that you can change those as well if you need to.

8) Jewellery
Jewellery must be kept to a plain wedding band and small stud earrings. Dangling earrings, bangles

• KEY POINT
Never, ever, chew gum or suck sweets whilst talking to, or working with, a client. This applies throughout the premises and, if you want to maintain the best impression with your clients, outside the premises as well.

• DID YOU KNOW?
Jewellery must be removed or covered if you are using electrical equipment.

and rings must be avoided at all times as they are unhygienic and may even injure your clients. Wrist watches should be removed and left in a safe place until the end of the day, but fob watches may be worn on your uniform.

CHECKLIST
This checklist provides a set of quick professional appearance checks that you can run through at the start of the day and before each client.
Before you meet your client check that:
- [ ] your personal hygiene is beyond question
- [ ] your uniform is spotless
- [ ] your hair is clean and neatly tied back from your face and collar
- [ ] your hands are freshly washed, and your nails are clean, neatly filed and unvarnished
- [ ] you are wearing appropriate make-up, and that it looks fresh and professionally applied
- [ ] you are not wearing heavy perfume
- [ ] your shoes are comfortable, your socks are clean and your tights are not holed or laddered
- [ ] your jewellery is, at most, a plain wedding band and/or a pair of stud earrings.

A word about punctuality
Your client is entitled to expect that when they arrive for their appointment their therapist will be ready and available to begin the treatment. If you are late and keep your client waiting this sends a clear message that you do not consider them to be your number one priority. Many clients, quite rightly, will feel upset and irritated if their treatment doesn't start on time.

Also, your employer will expect you to complete a treatment within a commercially acceptable time. For example, in most salons, it is considered to be commercially acceptable to provide a facial massage lasting for one hour, and the price set for that treatment will be based on the cost of one hour of the therapist's time, plus the cost of salon overheads such as lighting, heating, products used, and so on. If, though, the therapist spends longer than an hour providing a facial massage this will have an effect on the business – if fewer clients than expected are treated during the course of a day this means less money going into the till. This, in turn, will affect the employer's profits, and their ability to keep the business running successfully. In addition, clients often have busy schedules and plan carefully to fit a beauty treatment into an hour. If the therapist draws out the treatment so that it takes longer than an hour, this can have a knock-on effect on the client's plans for the rest of the day, and make them late for other appointments. What should have been a soothing and relaxing experience can, if it takes too long, turn into a frustrating and irritating event which spoils the remainder of the client's day. This is not good for the reputation of either the individual therapist, or the business.

Keeping to time is an important part of professionalism. If you find that you are regularly running late with clients – which means keeping the next client waiting – you need to reflect on why this is happening, so that you can address the problem. Some points that can help you keep to time are to make sure that you do not:

- draw appointments out by chatting too much
- forget to keep an eye on the clock
- overestimate how much you can do in a given time.

Always remember that, after one client leaves, you will need a few minutes in which to prepare the treatment room – and yourself – for the next client.

Endpoints
By the end of this topic, you should understand:

- being professional is about earning and keeping the trust of your clients
- your appearance should confirm to your clients that you are a professional therapist whose personal hygiene and presentation is beyond question
- you should know the time allocated for each treatment, and stick to it
- if, for any reason, you have to keep a client waiting make sure that you apologise sincerely, and assure them that the delay was unavoidable and will not happen again
- if you find that you are running late on appointments, think about why it happens, and address the issue so that the delay is not repeated.

TOPIC 2: PROVIDING A PROFESSIONAL ENVIRONMENT

As well as making sure that your own appearance is immaculate, it's vital to ensure that your treatment room, and everything in it, is spotlessly clean, neat, tidy and ready for the client's treatment. Needless to say, no client wants to find themselves in a treatment room which looks untidy or unhygienic. And, from the client's point of view, nothing appears less professional than settling down for a treatment only to find that the therapist has to leave the room to gather extra supplies or to find a piece of equipment that is in safe working order.

CHECKLIST

As one client leaves and before the next client arrives check that:

- the treatment room is spotlessly clean, neat and tidy
- you have opened windows to allow in fresh air, or used an air freshener, if necessary
- any bins are emptied before the next treatment
- your equipment trolley is clean
- you have sufficient supplies of all the products you need for the next treatment – e.g. fresh towels, tissues, cotton wool, products, etc.
- any equipment you intend to use is clean (and sterilised where necessary) and in perfect working order
- you have your client's records to hand or, for a new client, you have a new record card ready to be completed
- you have checked around the room to make sure that, in your professional opinion, everything is in order and ready for the next client.

The client will judge the quality of the service you provide on their complete experience with you. Even if the treatment you provide is perfectly satisfactory, if a client judges that some other aspect of the environment is unacceptable – for example, unhygienic or untidy – then they'll probably look around for another salon that provides a cleaner, more pleasant, more comfortable setting for their next treatment. In other words, you are quite likely to lose a client to another business.

Salon hygiene

Providing a hygienic environment is a duty we have to our clients. It is also, for your clients, an important criteria by which they will judge your services, and whether or not to return or to recommend you to their friends and acquaintances. Good salon hygiene is a continuous process that will, if carried out properly, ensure that all areas of the salon, and all equipment used within it, are clean and free from contamination.

Preventing infection means ensuring that micro-organisms (organisms that are so small they cannot be seen with the naked eye) such as bacteria, viruses and fungi do not have the opportunity to survive and multiply.

Bacteria

Bacteria are tiny, have a range of shapes – round, rod-like, or flagellate – and only about one thousandth of a millimetre across.

While bacteria can play a beneficial role in parts of the ecosystem, may even provide antibiotics, and can help with our digestion, they are a cause of diseases ranging in severity from upset stomachs to pneumonia, tuberculosis and typhoid fever.

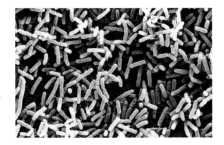

Viruses

Viruses are about a tenth the size of bacteria – indeed there is even one group, called bacteriophages, that feeds upon bacteria. They are responsible for some of the most devastating diseases of plants and animals. In humans, they are responsible for ailments from the common cold to herpes and HIV.

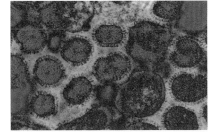

Fungi

While fungi can be seen (and enjoyed) as mushrooms, they are generally microscopic, and are another infectious organism that may affect us and our clients. They are responsible for the rising of our bread and the production of penicillin, but they are also the causes of ringworm, thrush, athlete's foot and fungal nail infections.

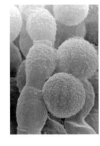 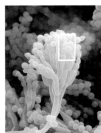

Type of infection	Characteristics	How it spreads	Examples
Bacterial infection	Caused by bacteria, which are single-celled micro-organisms	Bacteria reproduce at the site of the infection – skin, ear, throat, vagina etc.	Skin infections such as impetigo (staphylococcus pyogens) or acne (pro-pionibacterium acnes) Food poisoning such as salmonella
Viral infection	Caused by viruses, which are micro-organisms smaller than bacteria. Viral infections do not respond to treatment with antibiotics – penicillin etc.	Viruses reproduce inside human cells	Common cold Cold sore – herpes simplex, Chicken pox – herpes zoster, Wart – verrucae, Hepatitis A and B, HIV, which can lead to AIDS – Acquired Immune Deficiency Syndrome
Fungal infection	Caused by parasitic growth, which includes moulds, rusts, yeasts and mushrooms	Fungus is reproduced by spores	Ringworm – tinea pedis, capitis or corporus Thrush – candida albicans

PREVENTING INFECTION AND CONTAMINATION

A client can pick up an infection from equipment that has not been properly cleaned and sterilised, or from products that have deteriorated with age or have been contaminated by another client.

To prevent the spread of bacteria, viruses or fungus within your working environment it's vital that you take the utmost care to ensure thorough sterilisation and sanitisation. This will ensure that no cross-infection occurs between one client and another. A variety of sterilisation methods and techniques are available for use in the salon. Here are some of the most suitable.

Autoclave

An autoclave is an item of electrical equipment which is used to sterilise small metal items such as eyebrow tweezers and scissors. When water is heated at normal atmospheric pressure, it boils at 100 degrees centigrade. The autoclave heats water under pressure, which increases the temperature at which the water boils. At a pressure of fifteen pounds per square inch (psi) the boiling point of water is raised to over 120 degrees centigrade – a temperature at which good sterilisation can be achieved in twenty minutes. An autoclave, especially one with an automatic timer and a pressure gauge, is simple and effective to use and economical to run. Items to be sterilised must be capable of withstanding the heat in the autoclave, and this method is suitable for metal instruments. It is vital that all items are washed or wiped prior to being placed in the autoclave to ensure that all surfaces are free to be cleansed.

Disinfectant liquids and solutions

We are all familiar with the use of disinfectant liquids and solutions in the home, and appropriate products have a valuable role to play in the hygiene and safety of our salons. In salon use, a disinfectant must be effective, economical to use and inoffensive. Typical salon products are either chemical disinfectants that may require dilution according to their instructions for use, or alcohol-based disinfectants that may be used in the form of liquids, wipes, or gel-based hand washes. Examples include products such as Barbicide and Milton.

Unchecked, some germs spread so fast that they can double in number every half hour... so just one germ might become half a million in the space of a working day – hence the importance of regular and frequent attention to effective hygiene procedures in the salon.

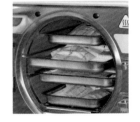

Before using any disinfectant product remember to:

- select an appropriate product for the use to which you are putting it
- clean before disinfecting
- follow the instructions
- wear appropriate safety equipment
- allow enough time for the product to work.

After use, remember that used products will be contaminated and no longer effective, and so should be disposed of carefully. Also bear in mind that some products, such as alcohol or gel hand cleansers may be flammable.

Ultraviolet radiation (UV)

Short wave ultraviolet radiation can be used to sanitise small items such as brushes and electrodes. The article to be sanitised is placed in a cabinet which must have already been cleansed. The UV radiation kills micro-organisms on the surface of the article. The UV radiation is only effective on the surface of items being sanitised (as it cannot pass through them) and, as light travels in straight lines, items must be turned during the process so that all surfaces are exposed to the light. The process takes roughly twenty minutes, and has the added benefit of not heating the item.

Chemical sterilisers

Liquid chemical sterilisers are plastic cabinets, usually with a perforated tray on their base. Most salon materials can be sterilised by cleaning and drying them thoroughly and then immersing them in the liquid chemical in the steriliser. After the time indicated on the manufacturer's instructions has elapsed (usually ten – thirty minutes), the items can be removed and should be thoroughly rinsed. It is very important to choose the correct chemical for your sterilisation needs. The chemical requires changing after the time specified by the manufacturer, usually about fourteen to twenty-eight days. Be very careful to avoid skin contact with the chemical.

Hot bead steriliser

Hot bead sterilisers are small and easy to use. They are suitable for sterilising small objects but not for brushes, plastic, sponge or glass. Tiny glass beads are contained in a protective insulated case and heated to 190–300°C (375–570°F) as indicated by the manufacturer. Sterilisation takes between one and ten minutes.

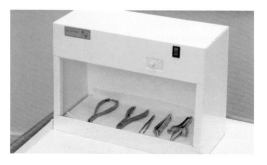

HOW INFECTIONS SPREAD

Infections are spread by touch, food, water droplets in the air, and through contact with cuts and grazes and other kinds of skin abrasions. Although it is almost impossible to create a completely sterile environment, you can reduce the risk of spreading infection by:

- not treating clients who have an obvious infection or, if the area infected is small, by avoiding it
- sterilising equipment
- disposing of waste safely
- maintaining the highest standards of hygiene.

CHECKLIST

Ways to ensure a professional level of salon hygiene:

- All hard surfaces – floors, worktops, trolleys, toilets, washbasins, etc – should be daily washed down with a disinfectant /sanitiser.
- Clean bed linen should be used for each client, or the treatment couch should be covered with clean couch roll for each new client.
- Clean towels must be provided for each client, and towels should be laundered daily.
- Clean towelling robes (if used) should be provided for each client.
- Towels, blankets, towelling robes etc. should be laundered daily and then stored in a closed cupboard or laundry bin.
- Waste bins should be emptied after each client and at the end of each day and disinfected.
- Broken glass or used needles should be disposed of in a sharps container as the contents are collected and professionally incinerated.
- If a client has any open wounds or abrasions on their skin you should avoid touching these areas, and should make sure that the wounds are covered with a plaster before the treatment starts. The same applies to the therapist.

Cross infection between clients can be prevented by:

- using disposable spatulas for waxing, etc.
- placing a small amount of product – blusher, foundation, cleanser, etc – onto a clean palette/spatula for each client; never using fingers to decant products
- not scraping back into the main container any product that has been in contact with either your hands or any part of the client.
- used cotton wool, tissues, etc should be immediately disposed of in a covered waste bin
- washing your hands thoroughly before and after every treatment, which is a must.

Thorough hand washing means:

- using an antibacterial soap or bactericidal gel and warm, running water.
- washing forearms, wrists, palms, backs of hands, fingers, between fingers and under fingernails .
- rubbing hands together for at least ten– fifteen seconds.
- using a clean towel or a disposable paper towel.

CHECKLIST
Health and hygiene terms you should know

- **Antiseptic:** a chemical used to reduce the growth of bacteria
- **Asepsis:** clean and free from bacteria
- **Disinfectant:** chemical used to destroy bacteria, not their spores
- **Non-pathogenic bacteria:** bacteria which are harmless or even beneficial to the human system, for example: lactobacillus acidophilus which is found in yogurt, and lactobacillus casei which is found in many cheeses
- **Pathogenic bacteria:** bacteria which are harmful and which cause diseases such as cholera, typhoid and tuberculosis
- **Sanitise:** make clean
- **Sepsis:** severe illness caused by overwhelming infection of the bloodstream by toxin-producing bacteria, which can originate anywhere in the body
- **Sterilise:** make clean and completely free from bacteria and their spores.

Endpoints
By the end of this topic, you should understand:

- infections caused by bacteria, viruses and fungi can easily spread from one client to another
- a client can pick up an infection from equipment that has not been properly cleaned and sterilised, or from products that have been contaminated by an infected client
- good salon hygiene is a continuous process
- thorough hand washing is essential to good hygiene as it will prevent the spread of any infection, and keep you and your clients safe.

TOPIC 3: PROFESSIONAL ENVIRONMENT

As a spa therapist good communication skills are at the heart of your ability to relate to your clients and to deal with them professionally. By using good communication skills you will encourage your client to relax in your care.

These skills include:
- asking the right kinds of questions
- listening with attention and interest
- being comfortable with silence
- using appropriate body language.

This, in turn, will contribute to their enjoyment of the treatment and should encourage them to return.

ASKING THE RIGHT KINDS OF QUESTIONS

Asking questions is one of the best ways of encouraging clients to communicate with you – giving you the information you need to treat them effectively.

When asking questions it's important to understand the difference between **closed** and **open** questions, so that you can ask the right kind of question at the appropriate time.

Closed questions are those to which your client will be able to give a short Yes or No answer.

Examples of closed questions include:

'Shall I open the window to let some air in?'

'Are you warm enough?'

'Would you like another blanket?'

'Have you had a facial massage before?'

Open questions can't be answered with a Yes or No. Open questions invite your client to provide information and to answer in detail. Examples of open questions include:

'What do you hope the treatment will achieve for you?'

'Tell me about how you sleep?'

'Which parts of your back are most stiff and sore?'

'Tell me about your diet?'

'How have you been feeling since the last treatment?'

● KEY POINT

Open questions are particularly useful when:

- you are meeting a client for the first time and need to take their history and complete their client record card (see Topic 7: Professional Record Keeping)

- you are talking to a client you have seen before and you want to find out how they responded to the last treatment you gave them and if there have been any changes, problems or improvements.

LISTENING WITH ATTENTION AND INTEREST

Listening to your clients with genuine interest and attention will put them at ease and will help to build a good professional relationship between you. On the other hand, not listening to your client may persuade them that:

1. You are not interested in them
2. You don't care whether or not the treatment you provide is appropriate for their needs
3. You do not have a professional attitude to the work you do.

Listening with attention and interest involves:

- being focused on your client throughout the time they are with you and concentrating on what they are saying
- listening without interrupting
- making eye contact with your client whilst they are speaking
- asking open questions to find out more
- remembering things your client has said to you so that at the next appointment you ask them about what they have told you – their holiday plans, family wedding, changes at work, new pet, and so on.

● DID YOU KNOW?

When a client hesitates before answering a question it is usually because they are trying to decide whether or not to tell you something important. Remember to give them time and encouragement... and to listen very carefully.

BEING COMFORTABLE WITH SILENCE

Some clients will enjoy talking throughout their treatment. They will regard the communication between you and them as an important part of the process, and they will happily chatter away about family and work and holidays and, probably, every other topic under the sun. Other clients, though, will regard their treatment time as a little oasis of peace and silence where they can simply relax and enjoy their therapy without having to make the effort to talk.

Once you have obtained any information necessary from the client, e.g. 'How have you been?'; 'Are you warm enough?'; 'Would you like another cushion under your knees?' If the client lapses into silence, don't feel that you need to make small-talk. This may be the only time during a busy working week when your client has the opportunity to completely relax and allow themselves to drift in peace and quiet. Don't spoil it for them.

• DID YOU KNOW?

Non-verbal communication is another name for body language.

USING APPROPRIATE BODY LANGUAGE

It is really important that you use appropriate body language with your clients, as this will put them at ease and reassure them that they are in the hands of a professional therapist.

Appropriate body language includes:
- smiling
- making eye contact
- sitting facing your client during conversation
- leaning forward slightly when talking to your client.

You also need to be able to read the body language of your client. For example, frowning, grimacing or raised eyebrows usually indicate that someone is irritated, uncomfortable or ill at ease.

• DID YOU KNOW?

The words you say are only a small part (7%) of the communication that takes place between you and another person. 38% of your message is communicated in how you say it, and a striking 55% is communicated through your body language.

Endpoints
By the end of this topic, you should understand:

- **the elements of good communication are being able to:**
- **– ask the right kinds of questions**
- **– listen with attention and interest**
- **– be comfortable with silence**
- **– use appropriate body language**
- **– make yourself clearly understood**
- **open questions are used to gather information, whereas closed questions are used to elicit a simple 'Yes' or 'No' answer**
- **listening with attention and interest will put your client at ease and make them feel valued and respected**
- **using positive and encouraging body language will help your client to relax and enjoy their treatment**
- **paying careful attention to your client's body language will help you to see when, even if they don't say anything, they are feeling uncomfortable or ill at ease.**

TOPIC 4:
PROFESSIONAL CLIENT CARE

Your clients have the right to expect a professional standard of care whenever they receive a treatment from you. Providing a professional standard of care involves:

- recognising contraindications
- taking account of your client's need for modesty and privacy
- not making false claims
- only providing those therapies in which you are fully trained and qualified
- not offering a diagnosis of any kind.

ITEC

Client Consultation Form – Body treatments

College Name:	Client Name:
College Number:	Address:
Student Name:	
Student Number:	Profession:
Date:	Tel. No: Day
	Eve

PERSONAL DETAILS

Age group: ☐ Under 20   ☐ 20–30   ☐ 30–40   ☐ 40–50   ☐ 50–60   ☐ 60+

Lifestyle: ☐ Active   ☐ Sedentary

Last visit to the doctor: ☐

GP Address:

No. of children (if applicable):

Date of last period (if applicable):

CONTRAINDICATIONS REQUIRING MEDICAL PERMISSION – in circumstances where medical permission cannot be obtained clients must give their informed consent in writing prior to treatment (select where/if appropriate):

- ☐ Pregnancy
- ☐ Cardiovascular conditions (thrombosis, phlebitis, hypertension, hypotension, heart conditions)
- ☐ Haemophilia
- ☐ Any condition already being treated by a GP or another complementary practitioner
- ☐ Medical oedema
- ☐ Osteoporosis
- ☐ Arthritis
- ☐ Nervous/Psychotic conditions
- ☐ Epilepsy
- ☐ Recent operations
- ☐ Diabetes
- ☐ Asthma
- ☐ Any dysfunction of the nervous system (e.g. Multiple sclerosis, Parkinson's disease, Motor neurone disease)
- ☐ Trapped/Pinched nerve (e.g. sciatica)
- ☐ Inflamed nerve
- ☐ Cancer
- ☐ Postural deformities
- ☐ Spastic conditions
- ☐ Kidney infections
- ☐ Whiplash
- ☐ Slipped disc
- ☐ Undiagnosed pain
- ☐ When taking prescribed medication
- ☐ Acute rheumatism

CONTRAINDICTIONS THAT RESTRICT TREATMENT (select where/if appropriate):

- ☐ Fever
- ☐ Contagious or infectious diseases
- ☐ Under the influence of recreational drugs or alcohol
- ☐ Diarrhoea and vomiting
- ☐ Skin diseases
- ☐ Undiagnosed lumps and bumps
- ☐ Localised swelling
- ☐ Inflammation
- ☐ Varicose veins
- ☐ Pregnancy (abdomen)
- ☐ Cuts
- ☐ Bruises
- ☐ Abrasions
- ☐ Scar tissues (2 years for major operation and 6 months for a small scar)
- ☐ Sunburn
- ☐ Hormonal implants
- ☐ Abdomen (first few days of menstruation depending how the client feels)
- ☐ Haematoma
- ☐ Hernia
- ☐ Recent fractures (minimum 3 months)
- ☐ Cervical spondylitis
- ☐ Gastric ulcers
- ☐ After a heavy meal
- ☐ Conditions affecting the neck
- ☐ After a heavy meal
- ☐ Conditions affecting the neck
- ☐ Any metal pins or plates
- ☐ Loss of skin sensation (test with tactile test)
- ☐ IUD (coil)
- ☐ Anaphylaxis
- ☐ Muscle fatigue
- ☐ Pacemaker
- ☐ Body piercing
- ☐ Excessive erthema

WRITTEN PERMISSION REQUIRED BY:

☐ GP/Specialist   ☐ Informed consent

Either of which should be attached to the consultation form.

RECOGNISING CONTRAINDICATIONS

A contraindication is a sign, signal or symptom that tells you that it would be unsafe to provide a particular kind of treatment or part of a treatment for a client:

- It might be unsafe for the client and could perhaps aggravate an existing illness.
- It might be unsafe for you and for everyone else in the salon.

Quite often the client will freely disclose, before the treatment starts, that they have a medical problem such as very high blood pressure or a heart condition. Many clients with all kinds of medical conditions benefit greatly from massage and other therapies that you are able to offer. But do make sure, in order to protect your client's health and safety, and your own reputation and the reputation of your employer, that you obtain approval prior to providing treatments.

Sometimes the client will not even be aware that there is a problem and it will only be when they have settled themselves onto the treatment couch that you notice something like recent scar tissue, severe bruising or what looks like a contagious skin infection.

Where there is a skin infection which could be contagious it's vital that you do not continue with the treatment as you could be at risk of:

- catching the infection
- spreading the infection throughout the salon.

However, it may only be necessary to avoid the area of infection not the whole person. Where you notice recent scar tissue, varicose veins, small cuts or abrasions, for example, it is fairly easy to work around these areas, making sure not to use any oils or other products or apply any pressure to the affected areas.

CONTRAINDICATIONS CAN BE CLASSIFIED INTO TWO DIFFERENT TYPES:

1) **Medical – your client has a medical condition, e.g. high blood pressure or diabetes.**
In these circumstances you need to obtain medical permission from the client's doctor before you can proceed safely with the treatment.
2) **Contraindications that may restrict the treatment.**
Beauty therapists should be able to understand and recognise those contraindications relating to beauty treatments requiring medical approval.

Where the client is unable to obtain such approval from a medical practitioner, the therapist needs to get 'informed consent' in writing from the client, which means that the client is made fully aware of the situation prior to giving any treatment for those contraindications that restrict treatment.

Contraindications for specific beauty treatments can be found in chapters 3, 4, 5, 6 & 8 of the book.

TAKING ACCOUNT OF YOUR CLIENT'S NEED FOR MODESTY AND PRIVACY

It is safe to say that, with few exceptions, most people (both men and women) have issues about one or more parts of their body.

For example, many women would like to have larger or smaller breasts, smaller waists, flatter tummies, thicker hair, smoother skin or daintier feet. In the same way, many men would like to be taller, more muscular or slimmer around the waist. The key point here is that, for some clients, the notion of removing their clothes and allowing a stranger to work on unclothed areas of their body may be quite daunting. It is therefore extremely important that you take account of your client's feelings throughout the treatment, and in particular ensure that your client's modesty is preserved at all times.

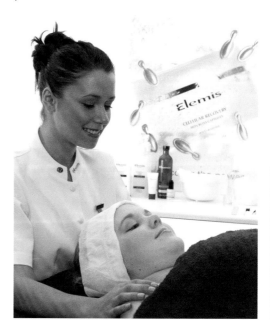

CHECKLIST

To ensure that your client's modesty is protected at all times:

- Before the treatment starts explain to a new client firstly which areas of the body you will be working on and secondly the garments they will need to remove. Also reassure them that they will be completely covered throughout the treatment apart from the small, specific area of the body that you will be working on at any one time.
- Allow your client to undress alone and in complete privacy, and make sure they have a clean, unworn robe to wear as they walk to the treatment couch.
- Once the client is settled on the treatment couch wrap them in a blanket and towels. This will preserve their modesty, keep them warm and also provide a feeling of being cosy, safe and completely covered up.
- When carrying out an intimate treatment such as an underarm or bikini wax, always provide a modesty towel and if, for example, you want the client to position protective tissues, always allow them to do this for themselves.
- Ensure that the client's privacy is protected at all times by making sure that no-one else can see into the treatment room. If, for some reason, another therapist enters the room during the treatment ensure that your client is fully covered so that their modesty is preserved whilst the other person is in the room. Even if the visitor is another therapist they are not your client's therapist and the client may feel embarrassed or uneasy.
- Make sure that your client has time and privacy to get dressed before your next client arrives.

Remember, your client is entitled to be treated with the utmost respect at all times – before, during and after their treatment.

NOT MAKING FALSE CLAIMS

As a professional you are required to work within the law. What this means for you, as a therapist, is that:

- if a manufacturer makes a misleading statement with regard to their product – for example, 'Will make you look 10 years younger' or 'Will burn away all unsightly fat overnight' and you repeat the misleading statement to a client, you may be liable to prosecution
- if you make false claims about pricing – e.g. 'This moisturiser is a great deal because we're offering it at £10 (half price) this week' when it actually cost £15 last week you could be liable to prosecution.

Imagine, for example, a client asks for a particular treatment and says 'I've heard this is really good and smoothes out all lines and wrinkles.' If this is not true you will only remain within the law if you, for example, either agree that it is a popular treatment, agree that you've heard some clients have had good results, or agree that the product smells nice, or is very pleasant to use (providing that all these statements are true), and that the client could certainly try it for themselves and see what they think of the results.

It is fine to say what you are aiming to achieve with your treatment or therapy, and what you hope might happen as a result. But it is really important not to make promises about the outcome the client should expect.

If you make unrealistic or untrue claims you are breaking the law and, almost certainly, your client will be disappointed and unhappy when your false promises fail to materialise.

To stay within the law you must NOT:

- supply information that is in any way untrue or misleading
- falsely describe or make false statements about products or services
- make false contrasts between previous prices and current prices
- claim that a product or service is being sold at 'half price' unless it has been offered at full price for at least 28 days prior to the 'half price' sale.

The Advertising Standards Authority states that adverts should be legal, decent, honest and truthful. This means that salon owners and their therapists should not make any false claims about any of the products, services or treatments provided to clients.

It's also important to be careful and diplomatic when discussing other therapists and other businesses. It's quite likely that, from time to time, a client will ask you for your opinion about another therapist, another salon, or even a therapy with which you are not familiar. Always make sure you say nothing that is discourteous or detrimental to another person or business. Making false or damaging comments is both unprofessional and dangerous as you could find yourself in court facing a case of libel.

ONLY PROVIDING THOSE THERAPIES IN WHICH YOU ARE FULLY TRAINED AND QUALIFIED WORKING WITHIN YOUR OWN SCOPE OF PRACTICE

As a professional it is vital that you recognise your role and its limits. From time to time a client may ask for, or you may feel tempted to offer, advice or treatment in an area in which you are not trained or qualified.

Don't go beyond your own limits. Always stick to what you know, and remember that you are in a relationship of trust with your client. If you go beyond the limits of what you can or should do, you are breaking that trust and may also be risking harm to your client. Always remember that if a client in your care is harmed then your own career and reputation may be damaged, possibly beyond repair.

In a situation where a client asks you for a treatment which you are not able to provide don't hesitate to refer them to a more experienced therapist. In these circumstances, always make sure that you have the client's permission before passing on any details of their treatment and health.

NOT OFFERING A DIAGNOSIS OF ANY KIND

In your career as a beauty therapist there will almost certainly be times when a client will ask 'Will you have a look at this … what do you think it is?' The client might be asking about a lump or a mole, a lesion, a patch of dry skin, a rash… there are any number of different possibilities.

No matter what you think or suspect, it's vital to remember that you are not trained or qualified to diagnose. Regardless of the circumstances do not offer your opinion but do suggest that the client consults their own doctor. You can do this without alarming the client by saying something like: 'To be honest, I really don't know what it is. If I were you I'd make an appointment to see your doctor or your practice nurse … they'll be able to have a look and tell you what it is.'.

Endpoints
By the end of this topic, you should understand:

■ a contraindication is a sign, signal or symptom that tells you it would be unsafe to provide a particular type or part of a treatment to a client

■ a contra-action is a sign or symptom that a client has responded unfavourably to a treatment or a product

■ when necessary, you should not hesitate to refer clients to their GP, practice nurse or another professional if you suspect they have a medical condition which needs attention

■ you should never offer a client a diagnosis, even if they ask. You are not trained or qualified to do this

■ you must always recommend only those treatments which are relevant and appropriate for the client

■ you must never offer treatments or advice outside the areas in which you are trained and qualified (scope of practice)

■ you must never make false claims for the treatments you provide, or the products you use

■ you must avoid making disrespectful or damaging comments about other therapies, therapists or salons.

TOPIC 5:
PROFESSIONAL HEALTH AND SAFETY

No matter where you work, under the law, both you and your employer have a number of health and safety responsibilities.

● DID YOU KNOW?

Your employer, regardless of the size or type of organisation where you work, has a responsibility to provide:

- a safe and healthy workplace which is kept in good condition
- equipment that is safe to use, e.g. scissors, computers, stepladders, tanning beds
- safe systems and procedures of work
- at least one person who is competent and trained to supervise health and safety at work.

You have a responsibility to:

- co-operate with your employer's health and safety requirements, procedures and policies
- follow safe systems of work – e.g. using equipment safely and following instructions for the use of products
- not interfere with or misuse any equipment or protective clothing provided by your employer
- take care of your own health and safety, and the health and safety of your work colleagues and your clients.

In large companies there may be very sophisticated first aid facilities with trained personnel and a dedicated first aid room. In most small businesses, though, it is considered sufficient to have:

- one person on the staff who is the appointed person who can take charge in an emergency situation – e.g. calling for the fire brigade, or an ambulance. The appointed person should receive Health and Safety Executive approved emergency first aid training, and also refresher first aid training every three years
- a first aid box which is kept well stocked with appropriate items
- an accident book in which all incidents can be carefully recorded.

Emergency situations involving work colleagues or clients can happen at any time. For example, someone at work might faint, burn or scald themselves, twist their ankle, have a nose bleed or start to bleed profusely from a cut, be stung by an insect, become dizzy, have an asthma attack or an epileptic fit, start to hyperventilate, fall into a diabetic coma, receive an electric shock or have an allergic reaction to a product you are using on them.

Even though you may not be the appointed person for dealing with accidents and first aid emergencies, it is vital that you understand what to do if an emergency situation occurs.

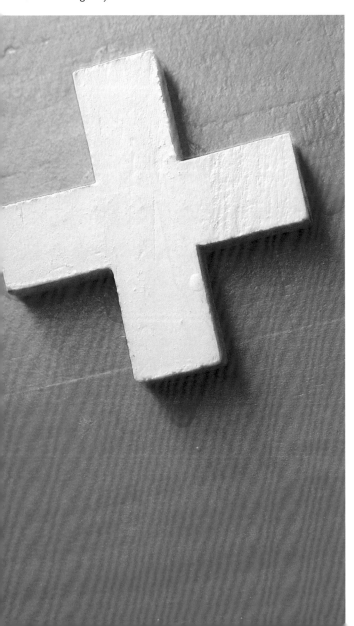

● DID YOU KNOW?

A risk assessment is the process of:
- regularly carrying out a careful examination of the workplace, equipment and work systems and procedures to identify hazards and potential hazards
- identifying and removing, or makingsafe, the hazards and then deciding whether or not any further action needs to be taken to eliminate similar hazards in the future
- taking further action as appropriate – maybe reorganising workspaces, arranging additional training for staff, changing working practices, etc.

A hazard is something that could cause harm to someone. Examples of hazards include:
- electrical plugs that have not been properly wired
- treatment couches that are in need of repair or replacement
- sharp scissors that are left lying around, and inappropriate disposal of sharp objects.

A risk is the chance that a hazard will cause harm to someone, for example:
- electrical plugs that have not been properly wired so that when you plug in the electrical appliance you receive a shock and, possibly, severe burns
- treatment couches that are in need of repair or replacement so that when a client lies down the couch gives way and collapses. The result being a very shocked client who may even sustain injuries such as a sprain or broken bone
- sharp scissors that are left lying around so that when a work colleague accidentally bumps into the couch where the scissors have been left, the scissors fly off and embed themselves in her arm.

CHECKLIST

Dealing with a first aid emergency
If someone at work, either a colleague or a client, becomes ill and appears to need medical help:

■ Immediately find the person who is the appointed person/first aider, and follow their instructions.
■ If the person who has been taken ill cannot, in your opinion, be safely left on their own, get someone else to find the appointed person.
■ If the appointed person is not in the building, call the emergency services.
■ Ask for the ambulance service and provide the information that the control officer on the other end of the line will ask for:
– your telephone number and your location
– the type and seriousness of the incident: e.g. someone has fainted, or scalded themselves very badly
– details of the person involved in the incident: sex, age, condition, etc.
■ If necessary, the control officer will pass messages on to the other emergency services such as the fire brigade and police.

● DID YOU KNOW?

You should never give another person any kind of medication – not even an aspirin or a paracetamol – as the person may be allergic to one or more of the ingredients and you could make matters much worse. Also, if you give medication to someone and it has a bad effect on them, you may be liable to prosecution.

THE RECOVERY POSITION

If someone is unconscious, there is a safe position which you can put them into which allows them to breathe easily and stops them choking on any vomit. This is called the recovery position.
In an emergency situation, if the appointed person isn't available, you may have to put a client or colleague into the recovery position. To do this:

■ check their airway is clear
■ check they are breathing
■ check they have a pulse.

CHECKLIST

How to put an adult into the recovery position

1) Position casualty's legs:
■ kneel beside casualty
■ straighten casualty's limbs
■ lift nearer leg at knee so it is fully bent upwards.

2) Position casualty's arms:
■ place casualty's nearer arm across chest
■ place farther arm at right angles to body.

3) Roll casualty into position:
■ roll casualty away from you onto side
■ keep leg at right angles, with knee touching ground to prevent casualty rolling onto their face.

4) The recovery position:
■ once in the recovery position, do not leave casualty unattended, and continue to check breathing and pulse regularly.

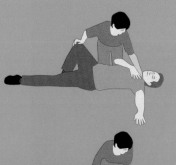
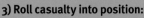
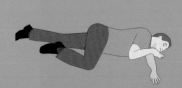

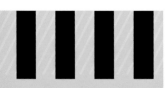

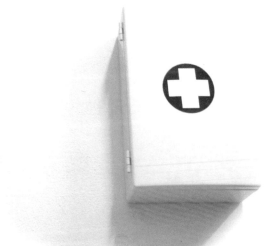

Warning

The casualty may have head or neck injuries.
It is therefore very important that:

■ you ensure the person's head and neck are
  supported at all times
■ you do not allow rotation between the
  head and spine
■ you do not tilt the head back if you suspect
  there may be a neck injury.

• KEY POINT

Even if you are not the appointed person at work
who is responsible for dealing with first aid
emergencies, it is important to have some basic
training. As you will be working with members
of the public we strongly urge you to complete a
recognised three-day training course.

THE FIRST AID KIT

There is no standard list of items which should
be included in a first aid kit, but the Health and
Safety Executive recommends the following as a
minimum:

■ a guidance card or leaflet which gives basic
  information about the most important
  emergency procedures
■ twenty individually wrapped sterile adhesive
  dressings (plasters in assorted sizes) which can
  be used for protecting cuts and other breaks in
  the skin
■ two sterile eye pads which can be used to cover
  the eye(s) following eye injuries
■ four individually wrapped triangular bandages
  (preferably sterile) which can be used as (1) a
  pad to stop bleeding; (2) as a sterile covering for
  large injuries such as burns or scalds; (3) as a
  bandage; (4) as a sling
■ six safety pins which can be used to secure
  bandages
■ six medium wound dressings (a sterile,
  unmedicated dressing pad with a bandage
  attached, size no 8 – approx 12 cm x 12 cm)
  which can be used to cover medium cuts and
  wounds
■ two large wound dressings (a sterile,
  unmedicated dressing pad with a bandage
  attached, size no 9 – approx 18 cm x 18 cm)
  which can be used to cover large cuts and
  wounds
■ one pair disposable gloves to be worn at all
  times when dealing with blood or other body
  fluids
■ IMPORTANT NOTE: A first aid kit should not
  contain medication of any kind such as over the
  counter pain killers and/or anti-inflammatories.

THE ACCIDENT BOOK

Every business which has ten or more people working in it is legally required to keep an accident book in which all accidents, no matter how small, are carefully recorded.

Even in smaller businesses it is a good idea to keep a note of any accidents involving yourself, your clients or your work colleagues, as you may need to provide details in the event of an insurance claim.

The accident book should contain details of:
- the date and time of the accident
- the nature of the accident, including where it happened
- a short description of any action taken, e.g. ambulance called and client taken to hospital; or cold compress applied and client sent home in a taxi
- the signature of the person who is responsible for filling in the accident book.

DEALING WITH A FIRE AT WORK

Your salon should be equipped with the correct kind of fire-fighting equipment. Fire extinguishers are available to deal with different kinds of fires.

The extinguishers you have in the salon will depend on:
- the type of equipment used in your workplace
- how many treatment rooms there are
- how many clients, on average, visit the salon each day.

Your employer will provide the correct type and number of extinguishers, but it's vital that you know which type of extinguisher to use if you need

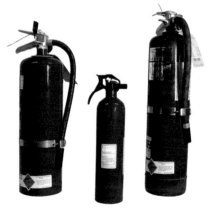

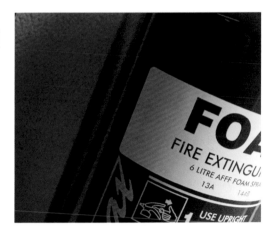

to use one should a fire should break out.

There are different types of fire extinguisher, for use on different types of fires and in different circumstances. So that they can be quickly and easily recognised in an emergency, they are colour-coded, with the most common colours and types being:
- Red (Water)
- Black (CO2)
- Blue (Dry Powder)
- Cream (Foam).

The table on page 2 lists some of the different types of fire extinguishers that you may come across, their uses, and importantly, when not to use a particular type of extinguisher. This is important as, for example, the use of a water extinguisher on:
- an electrical fire could result in an electric shock
- a burning liquid fire could cause the burning liquid to explode.

TYPES OF FIRE EXTINGUISHER

The types of extinguisher available, their recommended uses, and the colour-coding scheme may change from time to time, and you should keep up to date with current standards. The table on page 2 is adapted from www.fire.org.uk.

Type	Colour	Uses	Warnings
Water	Red	Fires involving solids – wood, cloth, paper, plastics, coal.	Do not use on burning fat or oil or on electrical appliances
Multi-purpose	Blue	Fires involving solids – wood, cloth, paper, plastics, coal. Liquids such as grease, fats, oil, paint, petrol, but not on chip or fat pan fires.	Do not use on chip or fat pan fires. Safe on live electrical equipment, although does not penetrate the spaces in equipment easily, and the fire may re-ignite. Does not cool the fire very well and care should be taken that the fire does not flare up again. Smouldering material in deep seated fires such as upholstery or bedding can cause the fire to start up again.
Standard dry powder	Blue	Liquids such as grease, fats, oil, paint, petrol, but not on chip or fat pan fires.	Do not use on chip or fat pan fires. Safe on live electrical equipment, although does not penetrate the spaces in equipment easily and the fire may re-ignite. Does not cool the fire very well and care should be taken that the fire does not re-ignite
AFFF (Aqueous film-forming foam) (multi-purpose)	Cream	Fires involving solids – wood, cloth, paper, plastics, coal. Liquids such as grease, fats, oil, paint, petrol, but not on chip or fat pan fires.	Do not use on chip or fat pan fires.
Foam	Cream	Limited number of liquid fires.	Do not use on chip or fat pan fires. Check the instructions for suitability of use on other fires involving liquids. These extinguishers are generally not recommended for home use.
Carbon Dioxide (CO2)	Black	Liquids such as grease, fats, oil, paint, petrol, but not on chip or fat pan fires	Do not use on chip or fat pan fires. This type of extinguisher does not cool the fire very well and the fire may start up again. Fumes from CO2 extinguishers can be harmful if used in confined spaces – ventilate the area well as soon as the fire has been controlled.
Fire blanket		Fires involving both solids and liquids. Good for small fires in clothing or chip pan fires if it completely covers the fire.	If the blanket does not completely cover the fire, it will not extinguish it.

EMERGENCY PROCEDURES IN THE EVENT OF A FIRE AT WORK

Employers are required, by law, to carry out a risk assessment, and to have a fire and evacuation procedure. By law, there must be at least one fire drill every year, which involves and includes everyone on the premises. Also, everyone must be fully informed and trained in what to do in the event of a fire.

You need to know:

- where the fire exits are in the building
- where the fire extinguishers are kept, and which kind of extinguisher to use for which kind of fire
- who to contact if you discover a fire, or if a fire breaks out where you are
- how to get your client safely out of the building
- where to gather – this is normally called the assembly point.

SAMPLE BUILDING EVACUATION PROCEDURE

If you discover a fire has broken out:

- sound the alarm
- call their local emergency services number
- if the fire is tiny and you feel confident that it can be safely, easily and quickly extinguished, use the appropriate fire extinguisher
- if you are at all unsure about whether or not you will be able to safely contain the fire with an extinguisher, your next priority is to get your client to safety
- if your client has undressed for their treatment make sure that they are provided with a robe and/or blankets and their own shoes.
- help your client to the nearest exit and take them to the designated assembly point
- wait at the assembly point with your client until the fire brigade arrives, and do not attempt to re-enter the building for any reason until you are told it is safe to do so.

Endpoints

By the end of this topic, you should understand:

- your employer has a legal responsibility to provide a safe and healthy workplace, and safe equipment, working practices and procedures
- you have a legal responsibility to co-operate with your employer's health and safety policies and procedures, to work safely, not misuse any equipment or protective clothing that is provided and to take care of the health and safety of yourself, your work colleagues and clients
- it is vital that you know what to do in the event of either an accident or a fire at work
- a hazard is something that could cause harm – a faulty plug, a frayed carpet or broken stepladders
- a risk is the chance that a hazard will cause harm – a faulty electric kettle blows up and someone receives an electric shock; or a client catches their toe in a piece of frayed carpet and falls, breaking their ankle
- all accidents at work must be recorded in an accident book. The entry must be signed by both the person who filled in the details in the accident book and the person who was actually involved in the accident.

TOPIC 6: SAFETY, RISK ASSESSMENT AND THE SALON

In the beauty salon, the main hazards to client and therapist include the:

- transmission of infectious diseases such as HIV or Hepatitis B
- use of chemicals
- safety of electrical equipment
- use of UV tanning equipment.

The next sections review some of the safety hazards that may be present in your salon, and suggest some ways of managing the risks they pose to staff and clients. This is not an exhaustive list, and will vary depending on the nature of your business and premises. The first step towards safety is a risk assessment. To begin assessing the risks in your environment, use the checklist at the end of this topic, and refer to some of the supporting material listed.

HYGIENE

There is risk of transmission of infection when using equipment and products on different clients.

Managing the risks

- Ensure 'hard' re-usable equipment such as tweezers and cuticle knives can be sterilised between use on clients.
- Remember that 'ultra-violet sterilisers' do not sterilise. Ultra violet light has sanitising properties only.
- Use disposable products where possible, e.g. sterile disposable needles for electrolysis and orange wood sticks for manicures, to avoid the need to sterilise equipment between treatments.
- Provide 'sharps' boxes for disposal of needles, blades, etc. These should be disposed of by a registered operator.
- Use techniques which prevent cross-contamination.
- Thoroughly cleanse brushes, sponges, towels, etc between uses.
- Contact your local council as you may need to register with them if you are carrying out skin piercing treatments.

ELECTROLYSIS

Under the local government rules, beauty salons that offer electrolysis may be required to register with their local authority and comply with relevant byelaws.

Managing the risks

The key points are to:

- use suitable equipment
- follow recommended methods
- have good standards of personal and environmental hygiene
- ensure staff are well-trained
- record all skin piercing treatments.

WAXING

The important issue with waxing is preventing cross-infection.

Managing the risks

- Hot and cool wax used for depilation should never be filtered and reused.
- Application should be with disposable spatulas that are then discarded.
- Observe good personal hygiene at all times.

HAZARDOUS SUBSTANCES

Some preparations and products used in salons may contain harmful substances that can cause skin or respiratory problems. Cleaning products can also be hazardous.

Managing the risks

- Make a list of all hazardous products used in the salon and obtain hazard data sheets from the manufacturers.
- Use the ECOSHH website at www.coshh-essentials.org.uk/ to carry out a COSHH assessment.
- Remember to include the risks from blood-borne viruses in your COSHH assessment.
- If you have a shower on the premises, include the risk of exposure to legionella bacteria from water.
- Make sure you are using the safest products available and that they comply with the Cosmetic Products (Safety) Regulations.
- Assess all new products before use.
- Store and use all products in accordance with the manufacturer's instructions.
- Dispose of surplus/out of date stock according to the manufacturer's guidelines.
- If dermatitis or asthma is detected action should be taken to minimise the problem by using barrier creams and gloves, improving ventilation, etc.
- Staff should be trained in the safe use of chemicals.

USE OF COSMETIC PRODUCTS IN SALONS

All cosmetic products used in salons must comply with the Cosmetic Products Regulations 1978 and when using such products you must:

- follow instructions carefully
- never mix products unless recommended by the manufacturer
- keep the original containers and ensure all containers are properly labelled
- maintain good standards of 'housekeeping' and personal hygiene
- use appropriate protective clothing
- not use them on clients with abrasions or irritated scalps
- store them in a dry place, at or below room temperature

- keep them away from naked flames (especially aerosols)
- dispose of unused mixtures and empty containers properly
- keep containers sealed when not in use.

For more guidance, contact the Hairdressing and Beauty Industry Authority at Oxford House, Sixth Avenue, Sky Business Park, Robin Hood Airport, Doncaster, DN9 3GG (tel: 0845 2 306080) or see their website www.habia.org for more details.

ASBESTOS

It is now illegal to use asbestos in the construction and refurbishment of premises, but much of that used in the past is still there.

While it is undamaged and undisturbed, there is little risk, but if it is disturbed or damaged asbestos fibres may be released into the air where they will be a danger to health if inhaled. The owners, occupiers or managers of non-domestic premises which may contain asbestos, have a legal duty to manage the risk or to co-operate with those who manage the risk.

Managing the risks

- Ensure an assessment is or has been carried out as to whether asbestos is or may be present in the premises and record the results.
- If an assessment shows asbestos is or may be present, the measures which are to be taken to manage the risk must be specified in a written plan.

ELECTRICAL EQUIPMENT

There are many different electrical appliances in use in beauty salons, and they are subjected to considerable wear and tear. Their portability and their proximity to water can create potentially hazardous situations.

Managing the risks

Appropriate precautions include establishing and maintaining an electrical equipment register and test/checking system, performing regular visual checks, fitting protective devices (such as a residual current device) to circuits to which portable hand tools are connected and ensuring correct earth bonding of pipework. A safe salon will:

- ensure electrical installations are maintained in a safe condition, and the state of fixed electrical installations inspected, tested and recorded by a qualified person every year
- have a system for regularly checking portable electrical equipment and an effective way of marking faulty equipment and preventing its use until repaired
- test all earthed appliances at periodic intervals
- keep a maintenance record for electrical equipment
- fit 30mA residual current devices (RCDs) to the main fuse board or to all sockets that hand-held equipment and sunbeds are connected to
- provide adequate sockets so that sockets are not overloaded through the use of adaptors
- ensure that all hot and cold water pipes are suitably bonded and earthed
- ensure that any mains gas pipework is suitably earthed.

SUNBEDS AND OTHER ULTRA VIOLET TANNING EQUIPMENT

Exposure to ultra violet light has associated health risks. A poorly-maintained sunbed may represent a risk of electric shock or fire. Precautions to manage risks will include the safe construction, installation and maintenance of the equipment, safe working practices that limit client exposure and the suitable training of therapists.

Managing the risks

- Make sure sunbeds have regular, recorded, services and maintenance and correct ventilation.
- Ensure sunbeds can be electrically isolated and there is an emergency cutout switch for the client's use.
- Ensure sunbeds have effective timers fitted, and that there is a way for the client to summon assistance in an emergency. In an emergency, the door of the sunbed room should be capable of being opened from the outside.
- Staff should understand the hazards associated with ultra violet light emitted by sunbeds and how to control their exposure to it.
- Potential customers should complete a medical

questionnaire before their first session.
- Keep clients' records, advise them of the health risks and the precautions they should take when using sunbeds. Instruct them on how the sunbed operates, its safety features and the maximum duration and number of visits they can make each year. Place advisory notices about safety and exposure in the sunbed room.
- When bulbs are replaced, make sure you inform clients to reduce exposure time and by how much.
- Provide washing facilities for use before the session.
- Provide suitable eye protection.
- Make sure that sunbeds and eye protection are thoroughly cleaned between uses.
- Introduce arrangements to deal with emergencies such as fainting.

FIRE

Many beauty products, particularly aerosols, are highly flammable and potentially explosive. Obstructions in fire exits can prevent escape and fuel fires.

Managing the risks

- Make regular checks to ensure all escape routes and fire exits are clear.
- Store cosmetic products, particularly aerosols, at or below room temperature, in a dry atmosphere, and away from naked flames or sources of heat
- Do not use gas heaters with a naked flame.
- Switch off and unplug all electrical appliances at night.
- Make sure employees understand what to do in the event of a fire.
- Heaters should be suitably located and fitted with guards to protect children and clients' clothing.

SLIPS, TRIPS AND FALLS

These may be caused by trailing cables or spilt liquids – most accidents happen when staff trip on leads or uneven floors, or are trying to reach items on high shelves. These hazards should either be prevented, in the case of trailing cables, or rectified promptly, in the case of spilt liquids.

Managing the risks

- Fasten cables and leads securely.
- Route cables overhead if possible.
- Keep passageways, workstations and stairs clear.
- Clean up spilt products immediately.
- Provide adequate lighting.
- Provide appropriate step ladders to reach anything not accessible from the ground.

Manual handling risks

Lifting and moving heavy items or working in poorly-designed spaces may cause back injury or muscular strain, known as musculoskeletal disorders (MSDs). These are by far the most common occupational ill-health problems in the UK, but:

- there are things that can be done to prevent MSDs
- the preventative measures are cost-effective
- all MSDs cannot be prevented, so prompt reporting and proper treatment are essential.

Managing the risks

- Avoid hazardous manual handling operations so far as reasonably practicable.
- Assess any hazardous manual handling operations that cannot be avoided.
- Reduce the risk of injury so far as reasonably practicable.

In the salon these can be addressed by:

- avoiding lifting items which are too heavy – use trolleys, lifts or other devices where possible.
- using proper lifting techniques.
- ensuring therapists have sufficient room to move around when working and provide chairs that can be adjusted to suit the client or therapist.

If there are risks to employees from manual handling, then a manual handling assessment should be carried out.

SAFETY AND RISK CHECKLIST FOR SPAS AND SALONS

Use the checklist below to initiate your risk assessment for your workplace. Remember that risks apply to clients, staff and members of the public.

Check	Yes	No
Have you identified areas of hazardous activity in your premises?		
Have you carried out risk assessments for each of the hazardous activities?		
Have you carried out any assessments required under COSHH 1994?		
Do you minimise exposure to hazardous substances through good working practices, good ventilation and staff training?		
Have you taken steps to prevent hand dermatitis, including staff training and the use of suitable gloves/skincare treatments?		
Have you registered any relevant skin piercing with the local council?		
Do you meet standards specified in byelaws governing skin piercing?		
Are the methods used for waxing such as to prevent the spread of infection?		
Is equipment so maintained and used to prevent the spread of infection?		
Do you have a register of all electrical equipment used?		
Is electrical equipment subject to a system of user checks and periodic inspection/testing as appropriate and are records kept?		
Are appropriate protective devices in place in the fixed electrical system?		
Is there a system in place to ensure safety in the use of UV tanning equipment?		

USEFUL SOURCES OF INFORMATION

The following may be useful references or sources of information relating to safety in the salon.

A guide to hygienic skin piercing

Public Health Laboratory Service, Communicable Disease Surveillance Centre,
1 Colindale Avenue, London, NW9 5EQ.

A short guide to managing asbestos in premises INDG 223 (rev3) Reprinted 12/04 C2000

HSE website or HSE's information line
0845 345 0055

Blood-borne viruses in the workplace: Guidance for employers and employees INDG 342 07/01 C1500

HSE website or HSE's information line
0845 345 0055

Code of Practice for Hygiene in Salons and Clinics

The Federation of Holistic Therapists, 38A Portsmouth Road, Woolston,
Southampton, Hampshire SO19 9AD
Tel: 01703 422695

Controlling health risks from the use of U/V Tanning Equipment Leaflet IND G 209

HSE website or HSE's information line
0845 345 0055

Health and Safety Implementation Pack for Hairdressers

Hairdressing and Beauty Industry Authority, 2nd Floor, Fraser House, Nether Hall Road, Doncaster, South Yorkshire DN1 2PH, Tel: 01302 380000.

Legionnaires' disease – a guide for employers IACL27(rev2) 02/09 C500

HSE website or HSE's information line
0845 345 0055

Manual Handling Assessment Charts Leaflet (MAC) INDG 383 08/03 C1000

HSE website or HSE's information line
0845 345 0055

Safety in the Salon

Hairdressing and Beauty Industry Authority, Oxford House, Sixth Avenue,
Sky Business Park, Robin Hood Airport, Doncaster, DN9 3GG – Tel: 0845 230 6080

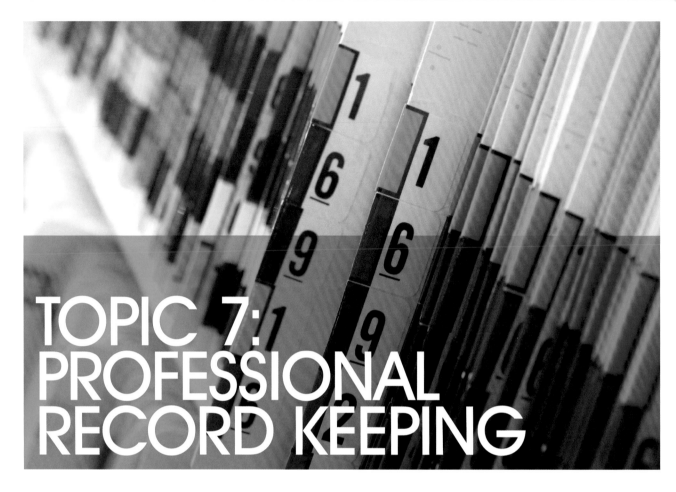

TOPIC 7: PROFESSIONAL RECORD KEEPING

WHY ARE CLIENT RECORDS IMPORTANT?

When you meet a client for the first time, it is important that you gain a clear picture of their health so you can identify which, if any, treatments are contraindicated, and also to determine what it is that the client is hoping to achieve.

For example, is the client suffering from work-related stress and hoping that their facial massage treatments will help them to relax and improve their sleep pattern? Or maybe, is the client reasonably fit and well, but hoping that a series of facials will help to improve their skin tone and restore skin elasticity?

CHECKLIST

The key benefits of keeping complete and accurate client records are:

- you know how to contact a client if you need to cancel or re-arrange an appointment, or if there is something you need to discuss with them

● DID YOU KNOW?

You are entitled to refuse to treat a client if they refuse to take a patch test. This is because, even if the client is willing to sign a waiver which makes it clear that they are willing to have the treatment without the test, this still leaves you, as the therapist, liable to a claim against you if the treatment causes problems for the client. This is because, professionally, you are responsible for carrying out the test.

- if there is a health emergency while the client is with you, you will know who to contact, e.g. their doctor or a relative
- getting to know the client and finding out about their likes, dislikes and what they hope the treatment will achieve for them
- you will have a written record of the client's health and medical history so that you will know which treatments are contraindicated. You can also keep a record as to whether or not the client has received approval from their doctor to go ahead with treatment, if the client has a medical condition that renders this approval necessary.
- if you are unable to keep an appointment with one of your clients, a colleague will have access to all the information they need so they can treat the client appropriately
- you can keep notes relating to which treatments the client has received, the outcomes, and whether or not the client wants to repeat the treatment again in the future.

TYPES OF RECORD CARDS

Client record cards tend to vary slightly from salon to salon, depending on the preferences of the person who owns the business, but they generally contain more or less the same basic information.

An example record card follows:

Client Consultation Form – Body treatments

College Name:	Client Name:
College Number:	Address:
Student Name:	
Student Number:	Profession:
Date:	Tel. No: Day
	Eve

PERSONAL DETAILS

Age group: ☐ Under 20 ☐ 20–30 ☐ 30–40 ☐ 40–50 ☐ 50–60 ☐ 60+
Lifestyle: ☐ Active ☐ Sedentary
Last visit to the doctor: ☐
GP Address:
No. of children (if applicable):
Date of last period (if applicable):

CONTRAINDICATIONS REQUIRING MEDICAL PERMISSION – in circumstances where medical permission cannot be obtained clients must give their informed consent in writing prior to treatment (select where/if appropriate):

☐ Pregnancy
☐ Cardiovascular conditions (thrombosis, phlebitis, hypertension, hypotension, heart conditions)
☐ Haemophilia
☐ Any condition already being treated by a GP or another complementary practitioner
☐ Medical oedema
☐ Osteoporosis
☐ Arthritis
☐ Nervous/Psychotic conditions
☐ Epilepsy
☐ Recent operations
☐ Diabetes
☐ Asthma

☐ Any dysfunction of the nervous system (e.g. Multiple sclerosis, Parkinson's disease, Motor neurone disease)
☐ Trapped/Pinched nerve (e.g. sciatica)
☐ Inflamed nerve
☐ Cancer
☐ Postural deformities
☐ Spastic conditions
☐ Kidney infections
☐ Whiplash
☐ Slipped disc
☐ Undiagnosed pain
☐ When taking prescribed medication
☐ Acute rheumatism

CONTRAINDICTIONS THAT RESTRICT TREATMENT (select where/if appropriate):

☐ Fever
☐ Contagious or infectious diseases
☐ Under the influence of recreational drugs or alcohol
☐ Diarrhoea and vomiting
☐ Skin diseases
☐ Undiagnosed lumps and bumps
☐ Localised swelling
☐ Inflammation
☐ Varicose veins
☐ Pregnancy (abdomen)
☐ Cuts
☐ Bruises
☐ Abrasions
☐ Scar tissues (2 years for major operation and 6 months for a small scar)
☐ Sunburn
☐ Hormonal implants

☐ Abdomen (first few days of menstruation depending how the client feels)
☐ Haematoma
☐ Hernia
☐ Recent fractures (minimum 3 months)
☐ Cervical spondylitis
☐ Gastric ulcers
☐ After a heavy meal
☐ Conditions affecting the neck
☐ After a heavy meal
☐ Conditions affecting the neck
☐ Any metal pins or plates
☐ Loss of skin sensation (test with tactile test)
☐ IUD (coil)
☐ Anaphylaxis
☐ Muscle fatigue
☐ Pacemaker
☐ Body piercing
☐ Excessive erthema

WRITTEN PERMISSION REQUIRED BY:
☐ GP/Specialist   ☐ Informed consent
Either of which should be attached to the consultation form.

An example record card

PROTECTING YOURSELF

In order to protect yourself against possible claims, make sure that you:

■ always complete a record card for a new client
■ update the card with appropriate details every time you provide a treatment for that client.

For some treatments the client will need to have an initial patch test to ensure that they are not allergic to any of the products used. It is vital that you record details of when the patch test was carried out, and the results. If, at some time in the future, the client complains about an allergic reaction you will have the results of the patch test so you can confirm that, at the time of the test, everything was fine.

Endpoints
By the end of this topic, you should understand:

■ a new record card should be completed for each new client, and should be carefully updated with all the relevant information every time the client receives a treatment

■ even if the client decides that it isn't necessary, or that they are willing to risk it, it is your responsibility to carry out a patch test where this is the normal routine for a treatment – for example eyelash or eyebrow tinting

■ if you do not carry out a patch test and the client develops an allergic reaction to a product you have used you, as the therapist, could be liable to a claim against you.

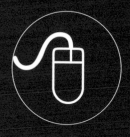

DON'T FORGET
TO LOGIN TO GAIN ACCESS TO YOUR **FREE** MULTI-MEDIA LEARNING RESOURCES

☐ **Over 40 minutes of instructional videos of all the key treatments**

☐ **Lesson plans and multiple choice and essay questions**

☐ **Interactive games and quizzes to help you to test your knowledge**

To login to use these resources visit
www.emspublishing.co.uk/spa and follow the onscreen instructions.

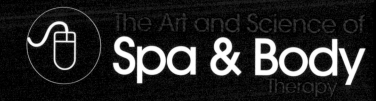

The Art and Science of
Spa & Body
Therapy

02

Body analysis

Body analysis will serve as a useful tool in many treatments you perform and is a key skill for a beauty therapist. Using knowledge of a client's body shape will enable you to recommend and treat on an individual basis, and correct for specific figure faults. Sometimes known as figure diagnosis, developing good body analysis skills will reward you throughout your practice and allow you to deliver tailored treatments. You will also earn the respect of your clients if you are able to correctly determine their body type and treat accordingly.

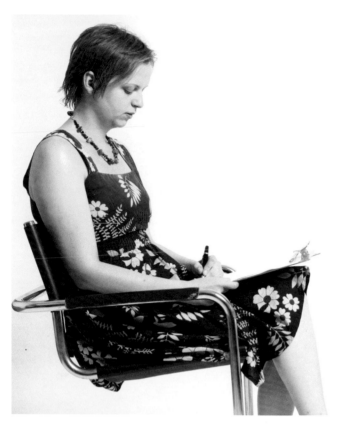
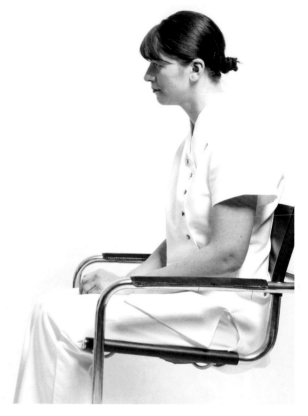

TOPIC 1: GATHERING BACKGROUND INFORMATION

When assessing a client's body it's important to remember that they may feel anxious or embarrassed. This could be due to perceptions about body shape, a figure fault for which they'd like to be treated, or discomfort at the possibility of taking clothes off in front of a stranger. A key part of treatment relies on your skill in putting clients at ease so they will give you honest information as well as taking accurate data and records.

EXPLAINING THE TREATMENT TO THE CLIENT

This is your golden opportunity to present yourself as a professional, calm any fears a client might have, and give them a comprehensive run-through of what they can expect from an analysis of their body.

1) Greeting

Greet your client with a warm handshake, make eye contact and use their name to welcome them to the consultation.

• KEY POINT

A client is far more likely to be open with you about personal details necessary for effective treatment if you are a patient and engaged listener.

2) Listening

Begin by asking the client what they're hoping to achieve from the analysis. Listen carefully. Turn your body to face the client and use nodding to encourage, particularly if they seem embarrassed or uncomfortable. Never interrupt, as often clients may pause on the brink of revealing something personal which is important to treatment.

3) Overview

Talk about the treatment in fairly broad terms, relating back to aspects which the client has mentioned they would like addressed. Explain in as much detail as possible exactly how the treatment would benefit them, but never promise results which cannot be delivered.

4) Areas not treated

If the client has mentioned any areas which would not benefit from the treatment be sure to communicate this to them, perhaps suggesting a different treatment for these aspects.

5) Step by step

If the client is happy to progress with the analysis, now is the time to explain what will happen throughout on a step by step basis.

It is particularly important to explain your reasons for weighing and measuring. Reassure your client, explain what can be achieved and lay-out the exact nature of the equipment which you will be using (weighing scales, tape measure etc).

• KEY POINT

Always protect the client's modesty, ensuring they are undressed for the minimal amount of time possible. Have clean robes on hand so they can undress in private but don't have to wait for you to re-enter in a state of undress.

6) Other aspects

Cover other specifics of the treatment such as:

a) The need to take a detailed assessment on paper before the other stages of treatment.

b) Where the treatment will be conducted – the treatment room or somewhere else.

c) Any clothing removal to be expected, and the form this will take. Explain they may be asked to remove their upper underwear, but lower underwear will remain in place.

d) How long the analysis will take.

e) What you hope can be achieved for them this session.

A word about client comfort

It can be very easy to forget that the client doesn't necessarily know what will happen during a given treatment. Particularly if you have administered it many times yourself. Always remember that a client's comfort is enhanced significantly if they know what to expect stage by stage. Verbal reassurance and guidance from the therapist is essential throughout the analysis.

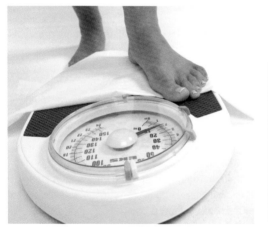

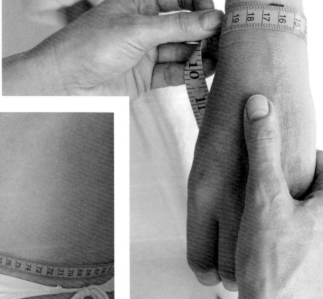

CHECKING CONSULTATION AND CONTRAINDICATIONS

After consulting with the client and explaining what they can expect you'll need to take professional records and notes. These will include any medical information and which parts of the body are to be treated as well the measurement aspect of body analysis. This is essential for the therapist to be able to carry out safe effective treatment, or even in some circumstances, decide whether to progress with treatment, at least for the moment.

Client Consultation Form – Body treatments

ITEC

College Name:	Client Name:
College Number:	Address:
Student Name:	
Student Number:	Profession:
Date:	Tel. No: Day
	Eve

PERSONAL DETAILS

Age group: ☐ Under 20   ☐ 20–30   ☐ 30–40   ☐ 40–50   ☐ 50–60   ☐ 60+
Lifestyle: ☐ Active   ☐ Sedentary
Last visit to the doctor: ☐
GP Address:
No. of children (if applicable):
Date of last period (if applicable):

CONTRAINDICATIONS REQUIRING MEDICAL PERMISSION – in circumstances where medical permission cannot be obtained clients must give their informed consent in writing prior to treatment (select where/if appropriate):

☐ Pregnancy
☐ Cardiovascular conditions (thrombosis, phlebitis, hypertension, hypotension, heart conditions)
☐ Haemophilia
☐ Any condition already being treated by a GP or another complementary practitioner
☐ Medical oedema
☐ Osteoporosis
☐ Arthritis
☐ Nervous/Psychotic conditions
☐ Epilepsy
☐ Recent operations
☐ Diabetes
☐ Asthma
☐ Chemotherapy
☐ Radiotherapy

☐ Any dysfunction of the nervous system (e.g. Multiple sclerosis, Parkinson's disease, Motor neurone disease)
☐ Bells Palsy
☐ Trapped/Pinched nerve (e.g. sciatica)
☐ Inflamed nerve
☐ Cancer
☐ Postural deformities
☐ Cervical spondylitis
☐ Spastic conditions
☐ Kidney infections
☐ Whiplash
☐ Slipped disc
☐ Undiagnosed pain
☐ When taking prescribed medication
☐ Acute rheumatism

CONTRAINDICTIONS THAT RESTRICT TREATMENT (select where/if appropriate):

☐ Fever
☐ Contagious or infectious diseases
☐ Under the influence of recreational drugs or alcohol
☐ Diarrhoea and vomiting
☐ Skin diseases
☐ Undiagnosed lumps and bumps
☐ Localised swelling
☐ Inflammation
☐ Varicose veins
☐ Pregnancy (abdomen)
☐ Cuts
☐ Bruises
☐ Abrasions
☐ Scar tissues (2 years for major operation and 6 months for a small scar)
☐ Sunburn

☐ Hormonal implants
☐ Menstruation (abdomen - first few days)
☐ Haematoma
☐ Hernia
☐ Recent fractures (minimum 3 months)
☐ Gastric ulcers
☐ After a heavy meal
☐ Conditions affecting the neck
☐ Any metal pins or plates
☐ Loss of skin sensation (test with tactile test)
☐ IUD (coil)
☐ Anaphylaxis
☐ Muscle fatigue
☐ Pacemaker
☐ Body piercing
☐ Excessive erythema

WRITTEN PERMISSION REQUIRED BY:

☐ GP/Specialist   ☐ Informed consent
Either of which should be attached to the consultation form.

CONTRAINDICATIONS

A contraindication is a condition which might prevent a client from receiving all or part of a treatment you're planning to administer. This might be a medical complaint but could also include a wide variety of issues from an emotional problem to an allergy. Be aware that people's bodies are different and contraindications which you may not expect could arise. In the event of a contraindication you may have to find a way to alter or adjust your treatment to work around the condition. Medical permission may sometimes be required. But you must also be prepared to cancel the treatment if the safety of your client would be at risk.

CHECKING FOR CONTRAINDICATIONS

Below are issues you should address when checking for contraindications.

Medical history

Clients may not immediately tell you about medical conditions, whilst others will freely share problems without being asked. A pre-existing condition could restrict a client's movement, making it difficult to assume a certain posture, or have other implications. Always find out if there is any pain, injury or other problem which you should know about.

Areas to be treated

Obtain thorough and detailed information about the specific areas which the client needs treated, and a history of any problems.

Physical condition

You will be able to take a more detailed analysis of a client's physical condition when you progress to more hands-on methods of analysis (see later in this chapter). However, much information can be obtained by talking with the client prior to this. With body analysis you'll need to take into account:

- Age
- Weight
- Size
- Muscle tone
- General health
- Specific issues

You may discover, for example, the client is very uncomfortable removing clothing, and be flexible to this requirement. Or that they have an aversion to being weighed by a stranger. It is important, however, that you give a truthful assessment, whilst respecting any emotional vulnerabilities.

● DID YOU KNOW?

Muscle tone changes with age, and an adult female loses around 22% of muscle mass between the ages of 30 and 70. This means older women tend to carry proportionally more fat.

Endpoints

By the end of this topic, you should understand:

- how to carry out a professional consultation and encourage clients to supply relevant information
- the need to explain fully to a client what to expect from a treatment
- the importance of respecting client modesty at all times
- what contraindications are
- how to check for contraindications.

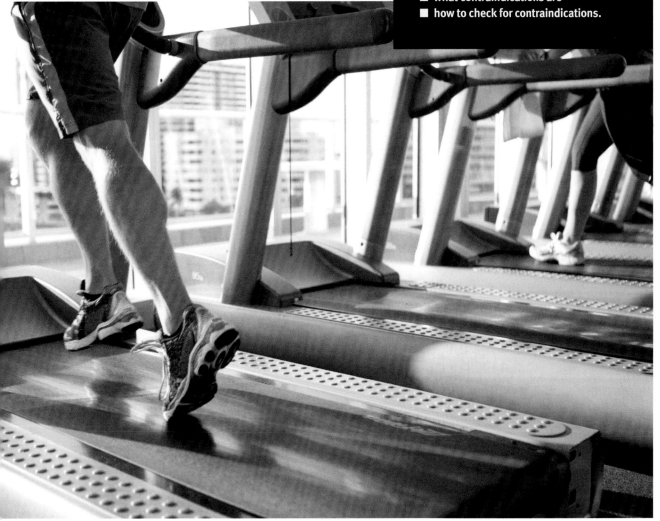

TOPIC 2: ASSESSMENT TECHNIQUES

During your consultations with clients you will be expected to keep detailed records and notes. It is vitally important for your own legal protection as a therapist that you obtain and confirm certain details with a signature to ensure you have taken due diligence with the health of your client. Crucially, however, on a day to day basis you will perform better services for your client with a good track record of their individual profile and progress.

CHECKLIST
When a client arrives for a consultation ensure you have to hand:
- [ ] a clip board
- [ ] several new pens and consultation forms ready to be filled out
- [ ] any details the client has already provided, such as name, age etc
- [ ] previous records if you have them
- [ ] any measuring equipment you will need, such as scales and tape measure, height stick, plumb line
- [ ] paper to take any extra notes.

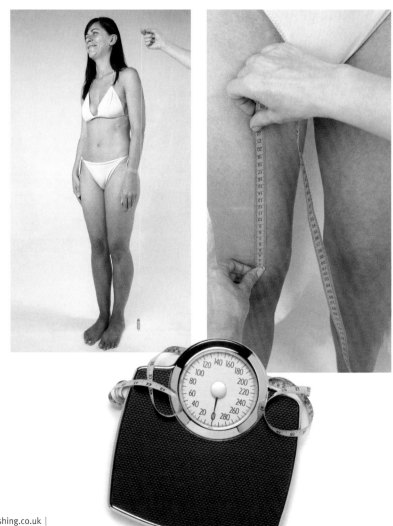

THE CONSULTATION FORM
Consultations forms will vary depending on where you practise. However they will all contain the same basic key points. Some of these will be related to legal protection such as disclosure of medical problems which might preclude treatment. For a sample consultation form, see page 40.

THE ASSESSMENT AREA
Ensuring an appropriate assessment area will make a significant difference to how comfortable the client feels about the diagnosis and future treatment. Whilst you would take the usual care

that such an area should be hygienic and tidy you should also:

- Use a dedicated treatment room to conduct the analysis if possible.
- Whilst relaxing low lighting is appropriate for many beauty treatments, good bright lighting is a better choice for body analysis.
- Have a clip board paper and/or the consultation form on hand to take notes as you make the assessment.
- Ensure equipment such as scales are out and ready to use.

VISUAL ASSESSMENT

At a later stage you will be using equipment and touch to ascertain information. Before you progress to this stage take as much data as you can using just your eyes. You may change some of these initial observations later, but they are a useful first assessment and after time you may find you can obtain as many useful details this way as when using more rigorous tests. Taking into account clothing you should look for:

SKIN TONE

Is the client's skin oily or dry? Aged, or youthful looking? Does the skin store fat in dimples, or it is smooth? Often you can gain an understanding as to the skin type on the whole body by seeing just the small portion outside clothing.

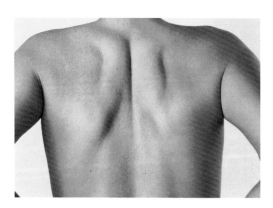

MUSCLE TONE

A firm and upright body usually suggests good muscle tone. You can often see from the appearance of any rigid contours whether the person has little body fat.

• KEY POINT

Write down any important details you notice as you carry out the analysis, rather than at the end. This way you won't miss any vital points.

• DID YOU KNOW?

The lymphatic system is as large and comprehensive as the blood vessel system. It interweaves with blood vessels carrying away toxic materials to be digested in the spleen and the lymph nodes.

TYPES OF FAT
Soft fat

This is adipose tissue found underneath the dermis of the skin and varies in thickness depending upon the condition and weight of the client. It is soft to the touch and tends to wobble. It is easily dispersed with diet and exercise and may overlay harder fat. It will also respond well to spa treatments designed for weight loss.
[sub-header] Hard fat
This fat often has a layer of soft fat overlaying it. It is more compact as it has been present for some time and as such is harder to loose or treat with spa treatments.

Trapped fat

This is hard and or soft fat which has become trapped within the muscle fibres and is very difficult to remove. It is most likely to occur in people who have at some time been extremely fit with highly toned muscles who have at some point ceased to continue their exercise regime. Muscle is re-placed with fat which then lodges in between the once very toned muscles fibres.

Cellulite

This is most commonly found in women particularly on the thighs and buttocks. It is thought to occur when interstitial fluid leaks out of damaged cells and becomes trapped between the fat cells making it very difficult to treat. It produces a very recognisable dimpled effect when the skin is in a natural state and not pinched. Diet and exercise may help as well as spa treatments that stimulate the circulation.

BODY TYPE

This will be covered in more detail in the next chapter, but clients can be roughly grouped into different body types which enables a therapist to make an informed decision about treatment. Basic body types used include mesomorph, ectomorph and endomorph.

FLUID RETENTION

Many people, particularly as they age, will accumulate fluid around their joints. This is known as fluid retention or 'oedema' (or 'edema in the USA). Pregnancy is also a major cause. The major reason is the lymphatic system which usually clears away excess fluid is less able to do this job effectively.

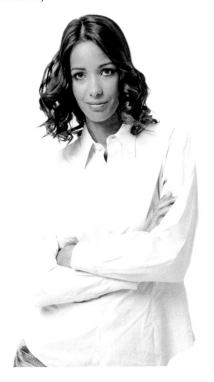

BODY LANGUAGE

This can give you vital clues both as to why a client may require certain treatment, but also how they feel about treatment. Overly constricted body language such as tense folded arms is your cue to do what you can do to relax the client.

POSTURE

This is explained in detail in Topic 4: Posture but a visual assessment can quickly take in some key postural imbalances and set the tone for later diagnosis.

RECORD KEEPING

During body analysis it is particularly important to keep proper records and notes. This will provide a meaningful history as to how a client has progressed and will act as a motivator throughout successive appointments.

You should treat your client records like a patient's medical records. Store them neatly, keep them in good order and ensure they are confidential. Good care of notes will assure clients you are taking their treatment seriously, and care about the long term outcome.

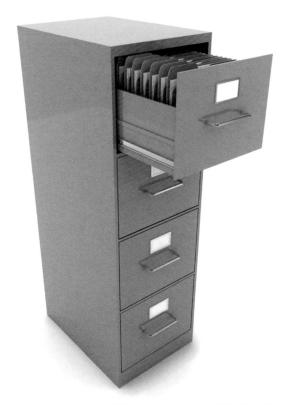

Endpoints

By the end of this topic, you should understand:

- ■ the importance of a carefully completed consultation form.
- ■ how to set up the right area for body analysis.
- ■ basics of visually observing different aspects of the figure.
- ■ good record keeping.

TOPIC 3: BODY TYPES

All clients are unique, but learning to group individuals into certain body type categories is very helpful for treatment. Not only will you gain an understanding of which treatments will work best for different body shapes, but you will know which longer term solutions will be most appropriate. Everyone falls roughly into three categories, or combinations based on these groups.

UNDERSTANDING AND EXPLAINING MORPHOLOGY

Morphology refers to the branch of biology which studies form and structure. In beauty therapy it is used to categorise individuals into three basic groups, each of which can tell us a lot about how an individual's body will react in different conditions.

These body types are determined by genetics, so whilst it is always possible to change the shape of a person's physique, it is not possible to alter their morphology category. It is possible, however, to use a knowledge of a client's morphology to deliver them the best treatment.

ENDOMORPH

This shape is your classic cuddly type, with a tendency to gain body fat. At their slimmest endomorphs have small frames with a very small waist. It is more likely, however, that you will encounter an endomorph carrying excess weight. As this type gains adipose tissue quite naturally, fat is deposited mostly around the hips and thighs to begin with and later the shoulders and abdomen.

An endomorph can retain a proportionally small waist into much higher weight gain than many, making them genetically predisposed to have healthier fat deposition. This is important, as it is

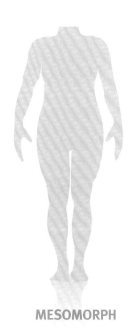

MESOMORPH

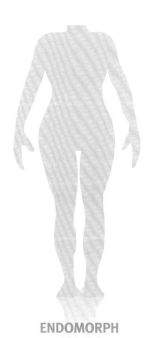

ENDOMORPH

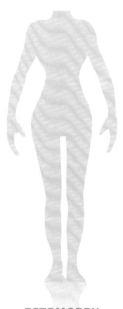

ECTOMORPH

easy to assume that every client of a larger size is an endomorph. In fact any body type can carry excess weight, and in order to correctly assess the endomorph proper attention needs to be paid to where fat is gained alongside additional factors.

Other factors to look out for:
- small hands and feet
- good natural flexibility
- good circulation
- short limbs and lower height in general
- soft skin and fine hair
- round physique.

Ectomorph

This is the body type which many women would choose for preference. Ectomorphs are slight framed, lean, and low in body fat. And whilst this means fewer feminine curves, this body type has long slim limbs and a tendency to put on neither muscle or body fat. The pure ectomorph can eat large amounts without gaining weight. The result is a physique which is fragile and delicate, with small joints. Many women ectomorphs feel their lack of body fat gives them an unfeminine appearance, whilst male ectomorphs may become frustrated with their lack of ability to acquire bulky muscle.

Other factors to look out for:
- long slim limbs lend a tall appearance
- small joints
- delicate body
- small bust
- lack of adipose tissue can make cellulite appear more pronounced.

Mesomorph

The mesomorph is usually the male body type of choice (if such types could be chosen), since it has a natural ability to build heavy bulky muscle. A mesomorph can put on muscle very easily, often in a very short amount of time, and for this reason this body type is also naturally very strong with very tough joints.

Mesomorphs appear athletic in build, with rounded limbs as a result of the muscle definition. This type will often choose to remain active and as long as they do so, will not have a problem with weight gain as muscle is a very powerful metabolic stimulator. The disadvantage to this type is that fat, if acquired, tends to lodge between the muscles which can very hard to get rid of. Fat also accumulates in the typical male pattern, tending to settle around the abdomen and spare the buttocks until a considerable amount is acquired.

Other factors to look out for:
- strong muscle tone
- hourglass shape (female), rectangular shape (men)
- good posture
- thick skin
- poor natural flexibility.

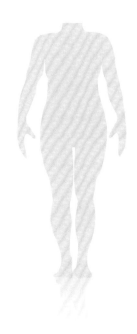

• KEY POINT

Whilst morphology is a helpful tool your client is still an individual. Be prepared that they might have a body shape which is new to your experience.

Combination

It is very likely that you will come across a body type which is some combination of the above types. So you may find a muscular mesomorph, for example, who acquires weight quickly like the endomorph, or a slim ectomorph with larger protruding joints. Current theory is that body types evolved to deal with different stages of evolution progression, from hunter gatherer to farmer, and as we're still evolving, new genetic combinations still occur.

OTHER FIGURE TYPES

Whilst morphology is a useful way to categorise body shapes an assessment of the fat deposition can also be used. This basically assesses where on the body fat is more likely to build up, and from this analysis, decisions can be made about effective treatments.

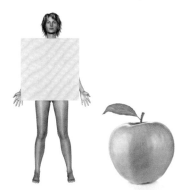

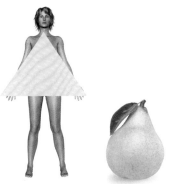

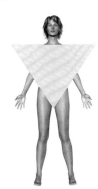

Square
(commonly known as apple)

Square types acquire weight around their middle areas, with fat settling mostly around the abdomen. Appearance at the extreme is 'apple on toothpicks' with a rounded bulky middle and slim legs and arms. This can be the result of genetics, but stress also plays a vital factor in signalling fat to settle around the waist. If the adrenal glands are constantly stimulated they will release emergency energy stores from the liver, which if unused (such as in exercise) will redeposit in the abdomen area as fat causing an apple shape. Treatment can play an important part in reducing stress and countering an apple physique.

Inverted triangle
(commonly known as pear)

This is the classic female fat distribution whereby fat settles around the hips and thighs. The appearance is pear shaped with rounded hips and thighs tapering to a smaller waist, and often small narrow shoulders. Pear-shaped fat distribution can be very stubborn to shift as the body tends to hang on to adipose tissue in this area. The reason for this is that as long as the waist remains small this is a perfectly health fat distribution, although aesthetically clients may feel differently.

Triangle

Triangle shaped individuals have broad shoulders and narrow hips, so the upper body can appear oversized – particularly on women. This body shape can be partially acquired through sports as many triangle shaped body types have a history of swimming or other activity which favours muscle acquisition around the shoulders.

● DID YOU KNOW?

Whilst fat around the middle is a more mobile kind which can enter the bloodstream and cause health problems, hip and thigh fat is relatively stable, acting as long term storage.

Endpoints

By the end of this topic, you should understand:

- reasons for categorising different body types
- the theory of morphology
- how to put morphology into practice
- how to define fat distribution.

TOPIC 4: POSTURE

With modern tendencies to spend long periods sitting, or walking in high heels with a heavy handbag, posture is often misaligned. And whilst it is easy to imagine that more involved treatments will have the greatest effect, posture education can be a powerful solution. Good posture can have a client appear pounds slimmer, with a firmer bust, taller frame and more commanding presence – all in a matter of seconds.

THE IMPORTANCE OF ASSESSING POSTURE

When a client comes to you seeking treatment it is vital that you suggest the most appropriate therapy at your command. For this reason postural assessment is essential to your practice. Any course of treatment designed to alter body shape will need to begin with a postural assessment.

This is especially important if a postural fault cannot be treated. Many clients will have acquired a stoop in the shoulder or may drop slightly on one side of the body – both faults which can be corrected relatively easily. Through assessing posture, however, you will ensure the client is not suffering from a fault which cannot be rectified or needs medical intervention, and may hinder treatment.

TREATMENT WILL NOT BE UNCOMFORTABLE

Postural assessment will highlight any discomforts in the body which can help the therapist adapt any treatment if necessary to accommodate them. It will also ensure that a treatment will not worsen an existing condition or cause harm.

EFFECTIVE TREATMENT IS SELECTED

Sometimes a postural imbalance may highlight the need for a different treatment than was initially suggested.

ADVICE FOR MINOR FAULTS CAN BE GIVEN

If a postural fault is minor the therapist can give basic corrective advice (see Topic 5: Postural problems), and thus prevent the problem from worsening for the client. Remember that if a client's posture is causing them pain or discomfort you should always refer them to a doctor.

WHAT CONSTITUTES GOOD POSTURE?

Most people can intuitively spot good posture when it is held in contrast with bad posture. But a subtle imbalance held over a number of years can often seem like quite a natural way for a person to hold their body.

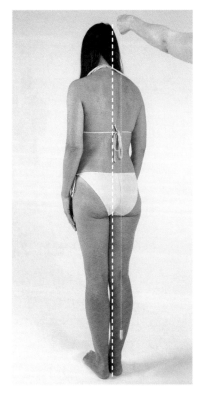

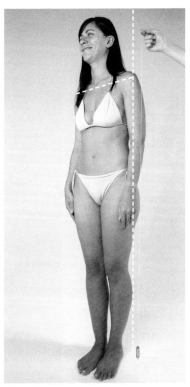

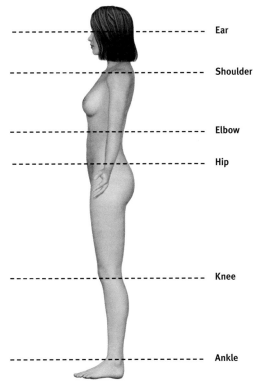

Ear

Shoulder

Elbow

Hip

Knee

Ankle

CHECKLIST

Points to look for in a good posture

- The head should not extend beyond the mid line (this is the imaginary 'straight line' you've drawn from ankles to crown).
- Relaxed arms should lie evenly at the sides.
- The distance between the scapula (shoulder blade) and spine should be even on both sides.
- Scapulas are positioned horizontally.
- Spine is straight.
- The back has a natural curve to the spine.
- Abdomen appears flat.
- Waist curves are level.
- Buttocks do no protrude abnormally.
- Legs are of equal length with forward facing knees.
- Body weight is evenly distributed.
- Feet should be forward and facing slight apart.

• KEY POINT

Few clients will come to you with good posture. But with only a few pointers and exercises you can radically change how a person holds themselves.

THE STRAIGHT LINE TECHNIQUE

Posture is all about straight lines. Look at the client in side profile and imagine a line running from their ankles straight up through their body. If this line goes through the middle of the body, up through the neck and out of the crown posture is good. Then assess them from a front angle and imagine a straight line running from shoulder to shoulder. This line should be exactly horizontal.

Endpoints

By the end of this topic, you should understand:

- the importance of posture to appearance
- how posture is relevant to beauty therapy
- how to assess good posture using the 'straight line' technique.

TOPIC 5: POSTURAL PROBLEMS

Whilst a straight upright posture is the ideal, most clients you'll see won't be holding their body in an ideal way. Most likely you will see small imbalances as well as common problems which can be relatively easily addressed. However, postural complaints can also build into more serious disorders, which whilst not a medical disorder as such, can cause discomfort or embarrassment for a client.

POSTURAL FAULTS

Any posture which deviates from good posture should ideally be corrected, but various structural complaints have also been defined as faults as a result of ongoing bad posture.

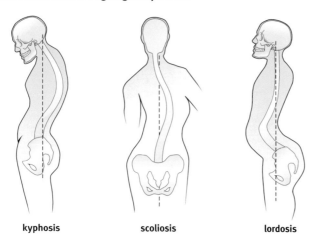

kyphosis   scoliosis   lordosis

Dowager's Hump
This condition is mostly seen on elderly people, in particular women. It results from a hunching posture which causes fatty deposits to be laid down on the back of the neck over time.

Exercise
Keeping the head and neck in a straight line is vital. But as the fatty deposits can force the neck down this can be difficult. The client should stand upright (fig.1), pushing the head and neck back, and hold for one second, release and repeat building up to longer times. They can also rotate the head gently from side to side (fig.2) whilst looking as far backwards as they can to exacerbate the movement.

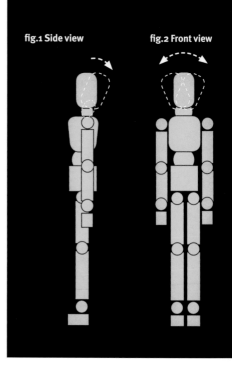

fig.1 Side view   fig.2 Front view

Winged Scapula

These are protruding shoulder blades caused by stretched pectoral muscles. They commonly result from carrying backpacks for prolonged periods, but excessive muscle building can also be a cause.

Exercise

You are aiming to tighten the pectoral muscles and loosen the adductor muscles in the back, pushing the scapula back into the right position. To counter this have the seated client (fig.3) hold small weights whilst bringing hands level with the ears and the elbows at 90 degrees. The client pulls the arms forward to bring the elbows and wrists to touch. Hold for two seconds, release and repeat for ten.

The cat stretch is also useful for opening the lower back (fig.4). Here the client is positioned on all fours, arching the back in a 'cat-like' posture and holding for two seconds before releasing.

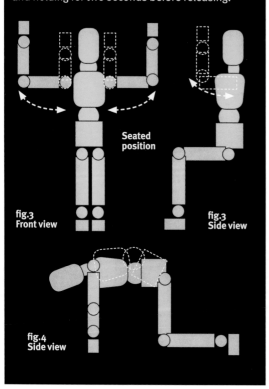

Seated position

fig.3 Front view

fig.3 Side view

fig.4 Side view

Kyphosis (rounded shoulders)

The opposite condition to winged scapula this is caused by over-tight pectoral muscles pulling the shoulders forward and down. This is a key correctional pose as it can lead to sagging breasts unsupported by stretched ligaments. You may see this in women who are self-conscious about height or bust size as well as those employed in jobs which see them regularly hunched forward.

Exercise

You are seeking to strengthen the scapula adductors (the muscles joining the shoulder blades). The client lies on the floor resting the forehead forward, arms extended in front with palms against the floor. Lift only the arms as high as possible from the floor (fig.5), hold for two seconds, relax and repeat for up to ten if possible.

Stretching the pectoral muscles is also helpful. This can be achieved using a seated exercise where the arms are lifted to keep forward facing palms level with the ears and elbows are at 90 degrees (fig.6) . Shoulders and arms are then pushed gently backwards, held for two seconds, released and the movement repeated up to ten times.

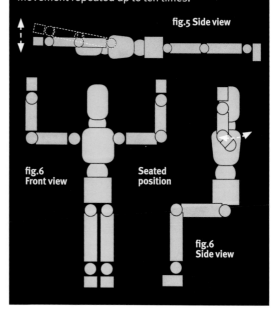

fig.5 Side view

fig.6 Front view

Seated position

fig.6 Side view

Lordosis (curved lumbar region)

This is the tightening of the lower back area, causing raised muscle around the spine and an unnaturally pronounced curve to the lumbar area. A common cause is high-heeled shoes as the body overcompensates for the forward tilt by leaning back into the spine. Likewise women who have been pregnant may also develop tight muscles in this region as a result of leaning back against the weight of their bump. Gymnasts and ballerinas can also be affected.

Exercise

The key here is to strengthen and tighten the abdominals, pulling the body forward. Stomach crunches are ideal as they do not put pressure on the spine. The client lays on their back, raising their knees to their chest and gently 'crunches' 30 degrees towards their bent knees (fig.7), pulling the stomach muscles in tight. Hold for two seconds and repeat for ten to begin with.

To tackle the lower back area the client lies on their back, pulling their knees hard into their chest (fig.8). Hold for ten seconds, release and repeat once more. Repeat the process one knee at a time, and then finish with both for a final ten seconds.

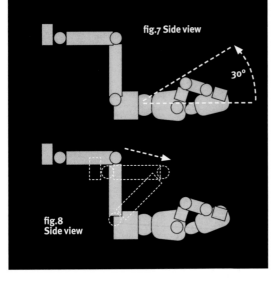

fig.7 Side view

30°

fig.8
Side view

Scoliosis (uneven spine)

This condition is the result of muscles on one side of the back being tight in one or more places. The result is the muscles pull the spine out of alignment into an S or C shape. Typical causes include carrying heavy bags on one side, or propping a baby on one hip. The waist line will be uneven and in some cases the pelvis tilts forward.

Exercise

Exercises should act to strengthen the muscles which have become stretched on one side. For uneven muscles higher in the back the client stands with feet shoulder distance apart and pushes down on the shoulder which is higher. Hold for ten seconds, release and repeat.

Lower muscles can be tightened by the client standing shoulder width apart, raising the arm on the lower side of the body with the opposite hand resting on the hip. Stretch up and over the head, hold for five seconds, release and repeat for ten building to twenty.

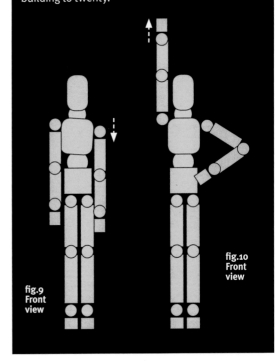

fig.9
Front
view

fig.10
Front
view

TOPIC 6:
MEASURING THE BODY

Whilst visually assessing a client can be a helpful way to assess figure and posture, physically measuring will supply a far richer source of data. Many clients assume that measurements will take the form of weighing scales, but this is only part of the data gathered. How weight relates to height and body shape is also vital to body analysis.

PREPARING THE CLIENT FOR MEASUREMENT

Upbeat tone
Many clients will be fearful and even distressed about what awaits them on the scales or within the measuring tape. Use your voice and body language to keep things light and cheerful. Try to avoid a 'medical' atmosphere which may make your client feel uncomfortable or under judgement.

Undressing
It is important that the client is undressed to their underwear for measurement, as clothes will impair your data. Follow the usual practice of allowing them to undress in private with a clean robe so they can await your return covered up.

Clean warm hands
Wash your hands in warm water and dry thoroughly to ensure they are not too cold, as you will be touching the client's bare skin.

Communication
Remember to continually come back to the client and check they are happy to proceed with the next measurement. Use a positive voice and no matter what measurements come back, always keep your tone light as you note down figures. It is very important that you never appear displeased as this may severely discomfort a client.

• KEY POINT
Measuring the body using equipment such as weighing scales and tape measures is also known as anthropometric testing – the estimation of the body size and weight.

WEIGHT
Whilst weight is not the only criteria used, it is a key indication of health and is useful in gauging client size. It is very important, however, that weight is not used as a primary indication, but rather a single piece of data in a wider picture.

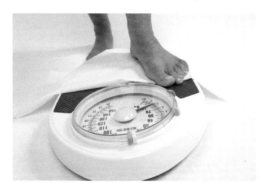

WEIGHING THE CLIENT
Ensure the weighing scales are on a flat hard surface. This is very important as a thick carpet can alter readings.

Have the client step onto the scales with their weight spread evenly, looking straight ahead and standing tall.

Read them the weight from the scales so they are not tempted to look down and alter their posture. Explain and note the weight in both stone/pounds and kilograms, as clients may have a preference for one style of measurement.

Reasons for fluctuating weight

- Different clothes. Clothes can weigh several pounds, so it is vital you weigh the client in underwear only.
- The client's body is not the only thing on the scales. You are also measuring whatever food and liquids they are carrying around on any given day. One litre of water weighs one kilo so this can make a significant difference to weight.
- For this reason the time of day can make a difference in weight, with clients tending to weigh more at certain times. If possible try to keep appointments to the same time each week.
- Menstruation, food allergies, food choices or certain medical disorders can cause fluid retention which will alter weight.
- Dehydration, on a hot summer's day for example or after exercise, can appear to reduce weight.
- Muscle acquisition through exercise will cause weight gain, even though fat may have been reduced.

Comparative fat and muscle weight

Per litre in volume muscle weighs 1.06kg, whilst fat weighs 0.9kg. This means that a client with a slimmer (and healthier) appearance may be heavier than a larger individual. More importantly for your practice it can also mean that a client who has been rigorously following a diet and exercise regime may have lost less weight than their appearance would suggest or even gained weight. It is crucial that you emphasise that inch loss is a far better indication of health, not to mention appearance to prevent a client becoming disheartened.

Comparative fat and water volume

As with muscle, water is slightly heavier than fat. One litre of water weighs one kilogram, and hydration is very important to health. It should be emphasised at all times that proper hydration with two or more litres of water a day is far more important than a few kilos difference on the scales.

• KEY POINT

Whilst two to four litres of water a day is optimum, never encourage your client to drink water in excess of this. Too much water (over a litre an hour) can throw-out the electrolyte balance in the body leading to very serious consequences including brain damage and death.

• DID YOU KNOW?

The medical term for fluid retention is oedema and can be caused by a number of reasons. Menstruation is a key reason for mild oedema, but medical problems such as kidney failure will lead to wide-spread fluid retention. Excess salt consumption can also cause fluid retention.

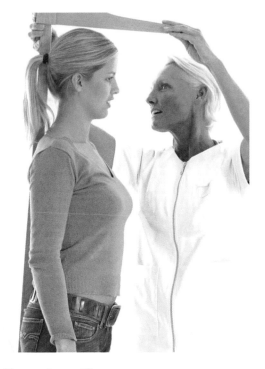

Measuring a Client

Taking a client's height measurement is relatively straight-forward but there are a few points to keep in mind.

Measure the client as they stand with their back against a wall – their buttocks and back of their head should be gently touching the wall.

Have them 'stand tall' with the shoulder back, closing the ankles and toes together, spine and neck straight.

The angle of the client's head can add or detract inches from their height. Have them fix their gaze levelly on the far wall and double check that the crown of their head is horizontal.

BODY MASS INDEX

The Body Mass Index is otherwise known as BMI. It is a medically used term to define weight to height ratios which are considered healthy. This means that numerous people could be the same weight, but based on their height their BMI will differ.

BMI has a range of around four to five stone within which a client can be considered a healthy weight. Many clients will be in this target range and yet still feel they would like to lose weight. This isn't necessarily an unhealthy attitude as a woman of average height could be twelve stone and still well within a healthy medical range, but for reasons of personal aesthetics would rather be a stone or so lighter.

If a client's goal is to fall on the lowest end of their BMI then this should be discouraged. Optimal health is perceived to be found in the middle of the scale by the medical profession.

CALCULATING BMI

Body Mass Index can be easily calculated by a medical chart:

For your professional development, however, you should also be able to calculate BMI based on weight and height measurements. Body Mass Index can be figured using either imperial (pounds and inches) or metric (kilos and centimetres).

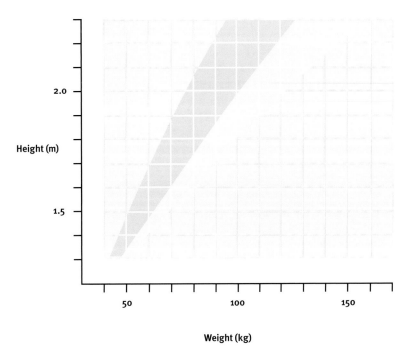

Height (m)

Weight (kg)

Metric Calculation

Client's weight in kilograms divided by height in metres squared.

BMI = (weight in kilograms)/(height in metres)^2

Method

First square the metres. This should be a number with a decimal point, so 166cm will be 1.66m. To 'square' means to multiply the height in metres by itself – so 1.66 x 1.66 in this example (the answer is 2.75).

Then divide the weight in kilograms by this figure – eg. 70kg / 2.75. The returned figure is 25.

• KEY POINT

The BMI index is a broad tool used by doctors. Whilst it can be useful for getting an indication of healthy weight, it must be used in conjunction with other measurements.

Imperial Calculation

Client's weight in pounds, multiplied by 703 (to give metric result) divided by inches squared.

BMI = (weight in pounds x 703)/(height in inches) ^{2}

Method

First square the inches. So 65.3 x 65.3 in this example (the answer is 4264).

Then multiply the pounds by 703 and divide the result by the inches squared (so 108262 / 4264). The returned figure is 25.

BMI Ranges	
BMI Number	**Health assessment**
‹20	Under weight
20-24.9	Normal
25-29.9	Slight over weight
30-39.9	Moderately obese
40+	Severely obese

• KEY POINT

The standard BMI measurement is in kilos so the imperial calculation is slightly more complicated as it converts pounds and inches to kilos and centimetres as well as working out BMI.

ESTIMATING HEALTHY SHAPE USING THE WAIST TO HIP RATIO (WHR)

Hip to waist ratio can offer the most accurate means of assessing the health and aesthetic appearance of a client. This is because where the fat settles on the body is often a better indication of physicality than how much adipose tissue is stored.

Two key sites of measurement are the hips and the waist.

■ Run a tape measure around the client's midsection at navel level.

■ Remind them to breathe normally, not holding the tummy in, and don't pull the tape so tight that it presses the skin down.

■ Note down both the centimetre and inch measurement.

■ Now repeat on the hipline to get the maximum hip measurement.

● DID YOU KNOW?

Many healthy young men have been turned away from joining the army because their BMI index suggests they are overweight, whilst in fact they are simply highly muscular. This shows that other measurements are necessary alongside BMI to ascertain health.

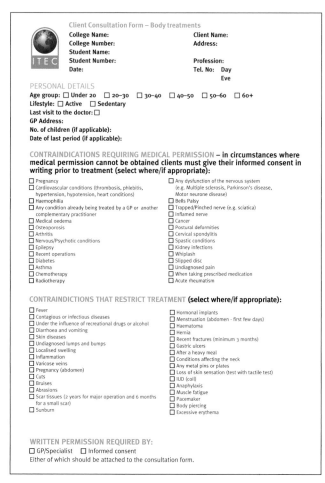

Client Consultation Form – Body treatments

College Name:
College Number:
Student Name:
Student Number:
Date:

Client Name:
Address:

Profession:
Tel. No: Day
         Eve

PERSONAL DETAILS

Age group: ☐ Under 20 ☐ 20–30 ☐ 30–40 ☐ 40–50 ☐ 50–60 ☐ 60+
Lifestyle: ☐ Active ☐ Sedentary
Last visit to the doctor: ☐
GP Address:
No. of children (if applicable):
Date of last period (if applicable):

CONTRAINDICATIONS REQUIRING MEDICAL PERMISSION – in circumstances where medical permission cannot be obtained clients must give their informed consent in writing prior to treatment (select where/if appropriate):

☐ Pregnancy
☐ Cardiovascular conditions (thrombosis, phlebitis, hypertension, hypotension, heart conditions)
☐ Haemophilia
☐ Any condition already being treated by a GP or another complementary practitioner
☐ Medical oedema
☐ Osteoporosis
☐ Arthritis
☐ Nervous/Psychotic conditions
☐ Epilepsy
☐ Recent operations
☐ Diabetes
☐ Asthma
☐ Chemotherapy
☐ Radiotherapy

☐ Any dysfunction of the nervous system (e.g. Multiple sclerosis, Parkinson's disease, Motor neurone disease)
☐ Bells Palsy
☐ Trapped/Pinched nerve (e.g. sciatica)
☐ Inflamed nerve
☐ Cancer
☐ Postural deformities
☐ Cervical spondylitis
☐ Spastic conditions
☐ Kidney infections
☐ Whiplash
☐ Slipped disc
☐ Undiagnosed pain
☐ When taking prescribed medication
☐ Acute rheumatism

CONTRAINDICTIONS THAT RESTRICT TREATMENT (select where/if appropriate):

☐ Fever
☐ Contagious or infectious diseases
☐ Under the influence of recreational drugs or alcohol
☐ Diarrhoea and vomiting
☐ Skin diseases
☐ Undiagnosed lumps and bumps
☐ Localised swelling
☐ Inflammation
☐ Varicose veins
☐ Pregnancy (abdomen)
☐ Cuts
☐ Bruises
☐ Abrasions
☐ Scar tissues (2 years for major operation and 6 months for a small scar)
☐ Sunburn

☐ Hormonal implants
☐ Menstruation (abdomen - first few days)
☐ Haematoma
☐ Hernia
☐ Recent fractures (minimum 3 months)
☐ Gastric ulcers
☐ After a heavy meal
☐ Conditions affecting the neck
☐ Any metal pins or plates
☐ Loss of skin sensation (test with tactile test)
☐ IUD (coil)
☐ Anaphylaxis
☐ Muscle fatigue
☐ Pacemaker
☐ Body piercing
☐ Excessive erythema

WRITTEN PERMISSION REQUIRED BY:

☐ GP/Specialist ☐ Informed consent
Either of which should be attached to the consultation form.

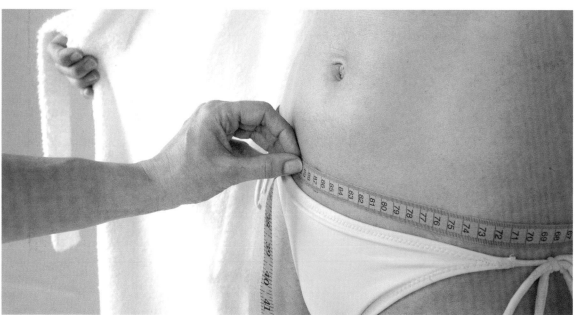

Calculating ratios

A healthy waist to hip ratio (WHR) has been defined as 0.7 or less for women and 0.9 or less for men. This figure is derived by dividing waist measurement by hip measurement.

A WHR of 0.7 or less for women and 0.9 or less for men may be considered healthy.

It makes no difference if this calculation is made in imperial or metric, but you must obviously use the same system of measurement for both waist and hip.

29" waist / 36" hip = 0.8

Or

73.66cm waist / 91.44cm hip = 0.8

• DID YOU KNOW?

Beauty icons through history such as the Venus de Milo, Marilyn Monroe and Audrey Hepburn all boast the 'ideal' 0.7 waist to hip ratio, even though they are markedly different weights and body types.

• KEY POINT

In a woman of healthy weight, a waist measurement of 35 inches or more indicates an unhealthy concentration of abdominal fat. Some research has shown that a measurement of 33 inches or more, no matter what the weight, increases health risks.

BODY FAT PERCENTAGE

A direct way of measuring fat is the measurement of skinfold thickness at key locations, using skin fold callipers.

Skinfold-based body fat estimation is sensitive to the type of caliper used, and technique. This method also only measures one type of fat: subcutaneous adipose tissue (fat under the skin). Skinfold thickness is determined at four sites:

- the triceps muscle
- biceps
- subscapular region
- supra-iliac region.

The single triceps skinfold thickness is sometimes used in medical surveys.

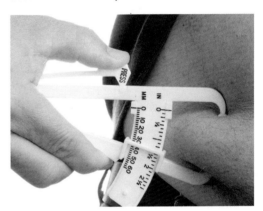

Endpoints

By the end of this topic, you should understand:

- the correct methods for weighing and measuring clients.
- the difference between weight acquired through fat deposits as opposed to water retention or muscle bulk.
- different techniques and methods for measuring clients.
- how to build a composite picture using various data.

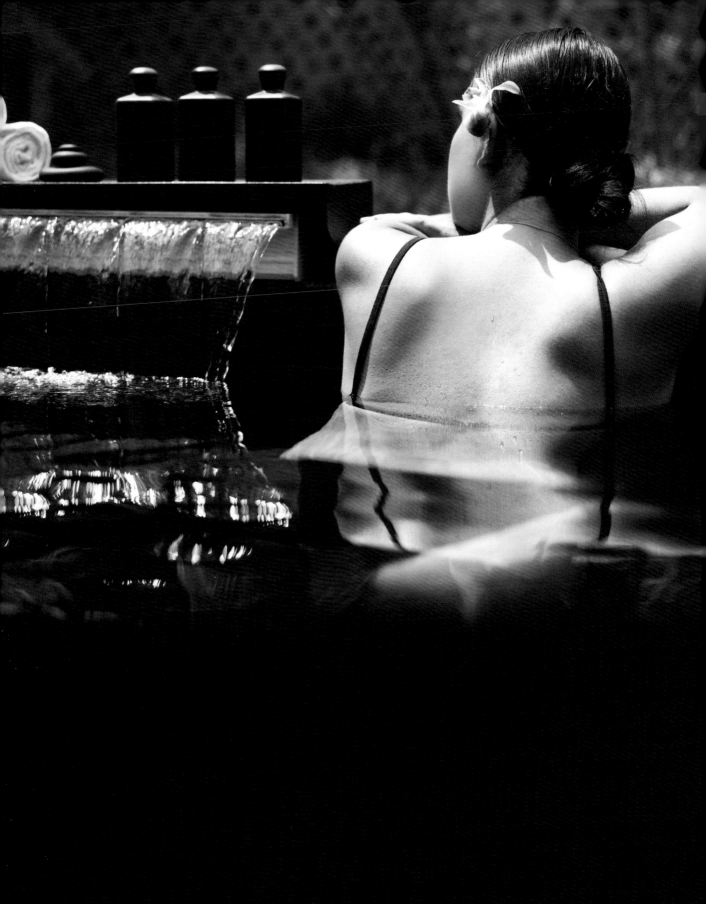

03

Exfoliation

Exfoliation is the process of sloughing away dead cells on the surface of the skin, encouraging better appearance and texture. There are many different ways of achieving this end, from mechanical (manual) methods to chemical creams and procedures, or combinations of the two. Each client is different and their skin type will determine how you choose an exfoliation technique.

A cross section of the skin

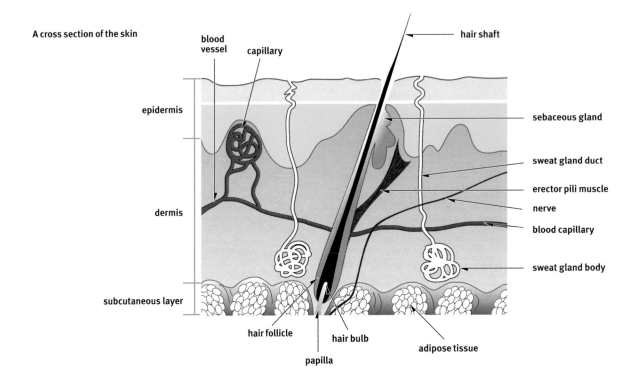

TOPIC 1: EXFOLIATION AND THE SKIN

Exfoliation works with existing structures of the skin to benefit cell growth and shedding, as well as clearing blocked pores.

The skin

The skin is the body's largest detoxification organ, and has numerous functions:

- protection and support of the body
- moderation of body temperature in cold or hot conditions
- sweat and excretion of toxins
- storage of water and fat
- synthesis of vitamin D.

The skin is the largest organ (group of tissues) in the body, both by weight and by surface area. It covers the whole body, is water-resistant, and has many functions including protecting and shaping the body. There are three layers: the epidermis, the dermis and the subcutaneous (hypodermis).

• KEY POINT

Exfoliation should always take place at the beginning of any treatment – NEVER when any heat treatment has taken place.

THE EPIDERMIS

The epidermis is the layer of skin that we can see. It varies in thickness depending on the part of the body it covers.

It is thickest on the soles of the feet and palms of the hand and thinnest on eyelids. The cells on the surface are constantly coming off (this is called desquamation) and being replaced from below as cells in the basal layer of the epidermis multiply and are pushed up to the surface. There is no blood supply to the epidermis, hardly any nerve supply and it receives nutrients and fluids from the lymphatic vessels in the dermis.

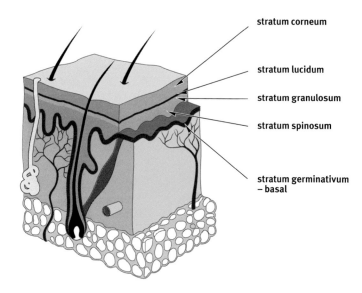

stratum corneum

stratum lucidum

stratum granulosum

stratum spinosum

stratum germinativum – basal

In total there are five layers in the epidermis:

1) **Stratum corneum – the surface:**
- is made up of hardened, flattened, dead, keratinised cells
- is constantly being shed through desquamation
- has an invisible cell membrane.

2) **Stratum lucidum – clear layer:**
- denucleated cells but not completely hard
- most easily visible under a microscope (only on palms and soles)
- cell membranes becoming visible.

3) **Stratum granulosum – granular layer:**
- cells have a distinct nucleus but cell membranes are dying
- contain granules which are visible in healing tissue after trauma.

4) **Stratum spinosum – prickle cell layer:**
- cells are living and membranes are intact; they have fibrils which interlock.

5) **Stratum germinativum – basal layer:**
- the primary site of cell division/reproduction (mitosis) in the skin
- cells are living. It is in this layer that cells are made. They take about 28–30 days to move up from here through the five layers of the epidermis before being shed.
- this layer contains a pigment known as melanin that gives skin its natural colour, whether red, yellow or black. Melanin is produced by cells called melanocytes.

THE DERMIS

The dermis is commonly known as the true skin. Unlike the epidermis, this layer is connected to the blood and lymph supply as well as the nerves. The dermis contains sweat and sebaceous glands, hair follicles and many living cells. It is made of connective tissue, mainly areolar tissue which is tough and elastic, and contains white collagen fibres and yellow elastic tissue known as elastin. Collagen plumps the skin and elastin keeps it supple and elastic. Both diminish with age.

The dermis contains eight main types of structure:

1) **Specialised cells:**
- fibroblasts: responsible for the production of areolar tissue, collagen and elastin. Fibroblasts can be damaged by ultraviolet light.
- mast cells: produce histamine as an allergic response and heparin, an anti-coagulant
- histiocytes: also produce histamine
- leucocytes: white blood cells which help to fight infection and disease.

2) **Nerve endings:**
- alert the brain and thus the body to heat, cold, pressure and pain
- part of the defence system of the body.

3) **Sweat glands which stretch from deep in the dermis to the outer layer of the epidermis. Sweat contains mainly water, urea and salts (mostly sodium chloride), and is produced by two kinds of gland:**
- eccrine: these excrete watery sweat and control body temperature, and are found all over the body, but especially on the palms of the hands and the soles of the feet.
- apocrine: these are found in the groin and axillae (armpits), and excrete a milky fluid which, when it mixes with bacteria on the surface of the skin, produces body odour.

4) **Hair follicles:**
- travel through the epidermis and the dermis.
- tiny muscles, called erector pili, are attached to each hair and help with the temperature control of the body by pulling the hair upright and trapping a layer of air – goose pimples.

5) **Sebaceous glands:**
- connected with hair follicles, and produce sebum, a fatty acid which keeps the skin moist

and which lubricates the hair shaft. They are therefore found in hairy areas, not on the palms of the hands or soles of the feet.

■ sweat and sebum combine on the surface of the skin to form the acid mantle, a protective shield which helps to control bacteria levels and prevents infections and disease and also acts as a natural moisturiser. The pH balance of the skin is 4.5–5.6 and this acid environment helps to prevent bacterial growth.

6) **Blood supply:**

■ a system of blood vessels including microscopic capillaries which are one cell thick.

7) **Lymphatic capillary:**

■ works in conjunction with the blood supply to carry waste products away from the area.

8) **Papilla:**

■ small conical projections at the base of the hair
■ contain blood vessels and nerves which supply the hair with nutrients.

THE SUBCUTANEOUS LAYER

This lies under the dermis and consists of a network of blood vessels, nerves, lymph and adipose tissue (fat cells). Its main function is to act as an insulator – both conserving the body's heat and acting as a shock absorber.

CELLS AND BODY TISSUE

■ Cells are the building blocks of our bodies. Many cells together make a piece of body tissue. There are four types of tissue: epithelial, connective, nervous and muscular.

Epithelial tissue (also known as epithelium)

There are two categories of epithelial tissue, simple and compound. Simple epithelium usually functions as a covering or lining for organs and vessels whereas compound provides external protection and internal elasticity. Goblet cells are often found in simple epithelium. These cells secrete mucus.

Simple epithelium

Simple epithelium consists of a single layer of cells attached to a basement membrane. There are four types: squamous or pavement, cuboidal, columnar and ciliated.

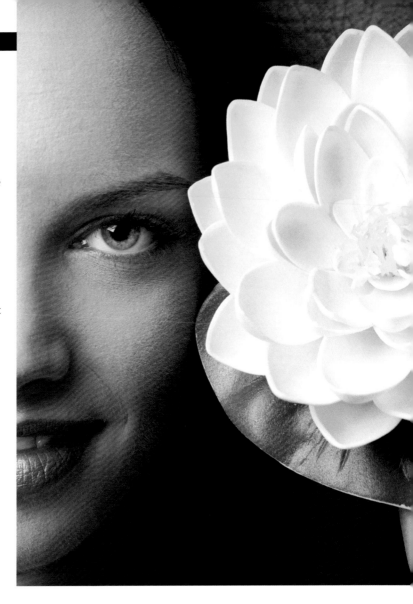

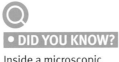
● DID YOU KNOW?

Inside a microscopic zygote is all the information needed to make a new human.

Squamous
Structure: single layer of flattened cells attached to a basement membrane.
Function: forms a smooth lining for the heart, blood and lymph vessels and alveoli of the lungs.

Cuboidal
Structure: single layer of cubeshaped cells attached to a basement membrane.
Function: forms lining of kidney tubules as well as some glands; can secrete substances and absorb them.

Columnar
Structure: single layer of tall, rectangular cells attached to a basement membrane; resilient.
Function: forms lining in very active parts of the body such as the stomach, intestines and urethra; some of the cells secrete mucus and some absorb mucus, depending on where they are in the body.

Ciliated

Structure: single layer of mostly columnar cells (sometimes combined with squamous or cuboidal cells) attached to a basement membrane. Tiny hair-like projections, or cilia, stick out from the cell membrane.

Function: the cilia work in waves, all moving together in the same direction. They help to remove mucus, foreign matter and debris, keeping passageways and linings clear. The respiratory system is lined with these cells.

Compound epithelium

Compound epithelium has many layers of cells and no basement membrane. It is formed from a combination of deep layers of columnar cells plus flatter cells towards the surface. It protects delicate parts of the body. There are two types: stratified and transitional.

Stratified

■ Keratinised (dry)

Structure: compound epithelium with dry surface cells; forms a dead layer e.g. hair, skin, nails. It is keratinised (i.e. the surface layer has dried out into keratin, a fibrous protein which creates a waterproof layer). Skin is stratified, keratinised, squamous epithelium.

Function: the keratinisation prevents deeper layers from drying out and protects them.

■ Non-keratinised (wet)

Structure: compound epithelium with wet surface cells e.g. inside mouth, lining of oesophagus, conjunctiva (mucous membrane) of eyes.

Function: provides lubrication.

Transitional

Structure: similar to stratified epithelium except that the surface cells are not flattened and thus can change shape when necessary; cube-shaped surface cells and deeper pear-shaped cells.

Function: found in organs that need waterproof and expandable lining e.g. bladder and ureterus.

Nervous tissue

Structure: arranged in bundles of fibres, composed of nerve cells and neuroglia. The cells have long fibrous processes. On a nerve cell these processes are called dendrites and axons. Function: capable of transmitting signals to and from the brain; protective.

Muscular tissue

There are three types of muscle tissue:

■ striated or voluntary
■ smooth or involuntary
■ cardiac.

Structure: all muscle is made of 75% water, 20% protein, 5% mineral salts, glycogen, glucose and fat.

Function:

skeletal: to help support and move the body;

smooth: to carry out involuntary functions, e.g. peristalsis;

cardiac: heart muscle to pump blood.

Connective tissue

Connective tissues are the supporting tissues of the body; they have mostly mechanical functions and connect more active tissues (like bones and muscles).

Structure: can be semi-solid, solid or liquid; can have fibres present or not.

Function: mainly mechanical connecting other more active tissues.

There are eight types:

1) Areolar

This is loose connective tissue, the most general connective tissue found in the human body.

Structure: semi-solid and permeable thus allowing fluids to pass through; it contains yellow elastic and white fibres as well as fibrocytes and mast cells which produce histamine (protection) and heparin (anticoagulant, prevents clotting).

Function: found all over the body connecting and supporting other tissues e.g. under the skin, between muscles, supporting blood vessels and nerves and in the alimentary canal.

2) Adipose

This is also known as fatty tissue.

Structure: made up of fat cells containing fat globules; found between muscle fibres and, with areolar tissue, under the skin giving the body a smooth, continuous outline; also found around the kidneys and the back of the eyes.

Function: protective and insulatory properties:

helps retain body heat because it is a poor conductor of heat; also a food reserve.

3) Lymphoid

Structure: semi-solid tissue; has some white fibres but not in bundles; lots of cells, the majority are lymphocytes and reticular cells which have a disease control function – the cell engulfs bacteria and destroys it.

Function: forms lymphatic system cells and blood cells and thus protects against disease; found in lymph nodes, thymus, the spleen, the tonsils, in the wall of the large intestine, the appendix and the glands of the small intestine.

4) Yellow elastic

Structure: mainly composed of elastic fibres and very few cells; this tissue is capable of considerable extension and recoil.

Function: to enable stretch and recoil, e.g. forms lung tissue, bronchi and trachea, arteries especially thelarge ones, stomach, bladder and any other organs that need to stretch and recoil.

5) White fibrous

Structure: strongly connective but not very elastic; consists mainly of closely packed bundles of collagen fibres with only a few cells in rows between the fibres; the fibres run in the same direction.

Function: connection and protection of parts of the body e.g. forms ligaments and the periosteum of bone; forms the outer protection of organs e.g. around the kidneys, the dura of the brain, the fascia of muscles and the tendons.

6) Bone

Structure: hardest structure in the body; two types, compact and cancellous – compact is dense bone for strength, cancellous for structure bearing and cellular development; composition of bone is 25% water, 30% organic material, 45% inorganic salts.

Function: to support and protect the body and all its organs, as well as produce cells in bone marrow.

7) Blood

Structure: fluid connective tissue, containing 45% cells and 55% plasma. Cell content is erythrocytes (red blood cells), leucocytes (white blood cells) and thrombocytes (platelets).

Function: to transport food and oxygen to all the cells of the body and to remove waste from them.

8) Cartilage

Structure: firm, tough tissue; solid and contains cells called chondrocytes. There are three types of cartilage:

Hyaline

Structure: bluish-white, smooth; chondrocyte cells are grouped together in nets in a solid matrix; particularly resilient.

Function: connecting and protecting; found on articular surfaces of joints, i.e. the parts of bones that form joints; forms costal cartilages and parts of the larynx, trachea and bronchi.

Yellow elastic cartilage

Structure: yellow elastic fibres running through a solid matrix. Contains fibrocyte and chondrocyte cells which lie between multi-directional fibres.

Function: flexibility; found in parts of the body that need to move freely, like the pinna (the cartilaginous part of the ear) and the epiglottis.

White fibrocartilage

Structure: white fibres closely packed in dense masses; contains chondrocite cells; extremely tough and slightly flexible.

Function: to absorb shock, e.g. it forms intervertebral discs as well as the semi-lunar cartilages, the shock absorbers positioned between the articulating surfaces of the knee joint bones; also found in hip and shoulder joint sockets.

Endpoints
By the end of this topic, you should understand:

- the different structures of skin
- how skin structure is affected by exfoliation
- the different tissue types made from cells.

TOPIC 2: REASONS FOR EXFOLIATION

There are a number of benefits to exfoliation, from the appearance of the skin at a surface level to skin health at a deeper level.

Improve skin texture and colour

Exfoliation acts to energise the process by which the body sheds dead cells. As the previous section shows, the surface of the skin is made from dead cells being shed on a continual basis (desquamation). Younger people's skin cells complete this process faster, meaning the top cells have been more recently generated and are less dried out.

By adding a manual aid to the process of skin shedding (desquamation), any sluggish activity will be increased, helping to generate the appearance of youthful skin by mimicking the fast cell growth of a young person.

• DID YOU KNOW?

When dealing with clients who have excess sebum production moisturising after exfoliation is essential. Stripping natural oils without replacing them can put over-active sebum production into overdrive.

Remove skin blockages

The sweat glands and hair follicles grow up through the dermis and open out through the epidermis. If skin growth is slow or a build up of dead cells on the surface is thick, these processes can be impaired.

In-grown hairs

Hair follicles can become blocked with skin cells, causing the hair to fold backwards onto itself and grow into a hard coil of hair. This can lead to an uncomfortable or painful raised bump of skin known as an in-grown hair. These can be freed by firm exfoliation, but sometimes need to be manually removed with tweezers. This is particularly important for depilatory procedures as the stripped hair follicle is enlarged after procedures such as waxing, making blockage and in-grown hairs more likely.

Sebaceous gland blockage

Oil glands which become blocked cause blackheads (comedones), or in inflamed conditions, spots or acne. This is a combination of excess build up of dirt and skin cells, and excess oil production. Exfoliation is very effective for blocked sebaceous glands.

Increase cellular regulation

Removing dead skin cells at the surface encourages renewed growth at lower levels of the skin. So whilst you're simply removing dead cells the body responds by speeding up cell generation leading to younger looking skin.

Increased absorption of creams

Skin cells are designed to be waterproof, and

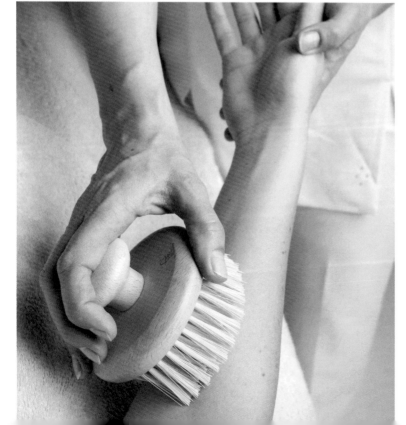

creams will not absorb into the dermis. However, sloughing away the tough dead cells on the epidermis will provide more surface area of younger fresher cells to absorb and benefit from creams.

Increase lymph circulation/detoxification

The skin is the body's largest detoxification organ, covering some two square metres in size. Toxic substances are mainly excreted through the sweat glands, but the skin can also be involved in manually stimulating the lymphatic system. This system takes toxic substances from the bloodstream and delivers them to the spleen where they are destroyed or inactivated.

As we will see later in Chapter 9: Massage techniques, lymph can be moved through manual manipulation of the body tissues, but exfoliation also helps speed up the removal of toxins.

Endpoints

By the end of this topic, you should understand:

- that exfoliation comes with a wide array of benefits
- main benefits of exfoliation, and how these can be explained to a client
- the impact of exfoliation on conditions such as cellulite
- effect of exfoliation on factors other than skin health, such as lymph and detoxification.

TOPIC 3: POSSIBLE CONTRAINDICATIONS FOR EXFOLIATION

Exfoliation is a non-invasive treatment. As it focuses on the skin, however, a variety of possible contraindications surrounding skin health must be observed. In particular therapists must be aware of contagious infections which can affect the skin.

Congenital

Congenital means skin conditions which are an ongoing complaint – something which the client is likely to have lived with for a long time. Often these type of skin problems flare up and are worsened by stress, so can be aided by relaxing beauty treatments.

Psoriasis

This is a condition caused by excess skin production, and is thought to be due to an overactive immune system. Some clients do find

that light exfoliation with a very mild scrub such as oatmeal can be beneficial, but others find it makes the condition worse. Active psoriasis should be contraindicated to exfoliation.

Blocked sweat glands

These are less common in cold countries as they tend to occur from a combination of excess sweating and dead skin cells. The resulting condition is known as 'prickly heat' and is an uncomfortable rash. Exfoliation should not be undertaken in the event of this condition.

Eczema

Like psoriasis, this is now thought to be due to an overactive immune system and causes sore inflamed skin. Active eczema should be contraindicated to exfoliation.

Dermatitis

This is a blanket term used to refer to any inflammation of the skin. Do not exfoliate skin which is sore, cracked or inflamed.

Inflamed varicose veins

Whilst pronounced varicose veins can often be a good candidate for gentle stimulation by exfoliation, you should not exfoliate directly over sore or inflamed veins. Check with your client if you are unsure.

Infestations

Infestations refer to conditions where a parasite has taken residence. This means creatures sometimes too small to be seen with the human eye are living in or under the skin. Whilst you may not be able to see the parasite itself, however, you will be able to see physical signs (rash, inflamed skin) or symptoms (itching) of the infestation.

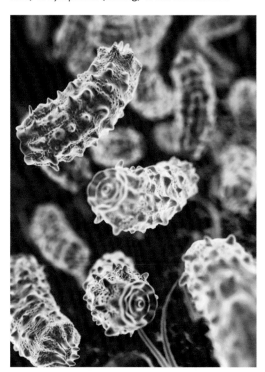

● KEY POINT

Many skin conditions mean parts of the client's body are not suitable for exfoliation. But unless the condition is widespread (or infectious) you may be able to work around or restrict treatment of problem areas. This is why a key therapeutic skill is listening and communicating with your client.

Scabies

Scabies is an infestation of microscopic mites which burrow under the skin, causing a raised itchy rash all over the body. Scabies is very infectious and no attempt should be made to treat a patient suffering from this condition. Additionally, any area in which an infected person has been in contact should be thoroughly cleansed.

Lice

A body lice infestation is extremely rare in the UK, and it is highly unlikely that you will encounter this condition as a therapist as they thrive only on very unclean skin. Head lice, however are reasonably common, particularly amongst those who have contact with children. These can be identified by small white eggs in the hair and itching. It is easily treated by over-the-counter remedies.

Head lice are infectious, but only if infected hair is brought into direct contact with another scalp. If you notice an infection, tactfully alert the client and ensure any areas in which their head has been in contact has been treated. You may also consider treating your own hair if there is a risk you have been contaminated.

Viral

Viral infections enter the cells of the body, and burrow into the nucleus, where they can hijack the body's own mechanisms to make new versions of themselves. Even after an infection has taken hold and been overcome by the immune system, the virus still lies hidden in the nucleus. They then appear to be able to sense when the body is under stress (and therefore in weakened immunity) and use this time to reproduce and re-infect.

As viruses are long-lived in this way, and can reoccur throughout a lifetime, they are particularly unpleasant conditions to contract, and great care should be taken to avoid contamination and infection.

Warts

Warts are a viral infection, which the body usually rids itself of after a lengthy period of time. They are infectious, and you should avoid treating areas of the body with warts.

Herpes Simplex

Otherwise known as cold-sores, herpes is extremely common and it is estimated 60% of people carry the virus. As long as you are not treating the facial area, treatments can be carried out on a client with cold sores, but you should take extra hygiene precautions and avoid touching your own face during treatment.

Fungal

Fungal infections are usually localised to one part of the body, with the feet being particularly vulnerable. They can be treated and cleared up permanently, but are infectious and care should be taken to avoid contamination.

Fungal problems usually occur when an imbalance of conditions such as acidity or yeast allow fungus to grow out of control, overwhelming the body's natural mechanisms of restoring normal conditions.

Bacterial infections

This is a general term, but usually applies to an infection of the feet. It is characterised by flaky white skin around the toes, scaly, flaking toenails, yellowing toenails or distortions of the toenails as the bacteria raises them from the toes. Generally speaking it is possible to treat clients with foot disorders as long as a pair of socks are worn.

Ringworm

Ringworm is a fungal infection which grows into a raised red ring. It can also form other shapes, but is generally characterised by a line of raised skin. It is infectious, and contact should be avoided until the condition has been treated by a medical professional.

Skin injury

Any kind of injury from a small scratch or bruise to a more serious abrasion should not be exfoliated, or be subject to treatment from other creams or treatments such as fake tan.

Endpoints

By the end of this topic, you should understand:

- that exfoliation may have possible contraindications
- the main forms these will take – bacterial, viral, fungal, and parasitic (infestations).

TOPIC 4: EXFOLIATION METHODS

Exfoliation can vary in intensity and a wide array of products and methods can be used. Depending on the client's skin type you'll want to choose a treatment to suit their individual needs.

Manual methods

These refer to exfoliation methods which physically remove the dead skin cells from the surface of the skin. On the most basic level, even rubbing the skin with a clean towel will count as some degree of exfoliation, but therapists use brushes, scrubs and other tools to achieve professional results.

Before undertaking exfoliation of the whole body, you must check that the client has consented to the areas you will be treating.

Dry-brushing

This is one of the most traditional methods associated with exfoliation, and uses a long handled brush of natural bristles.

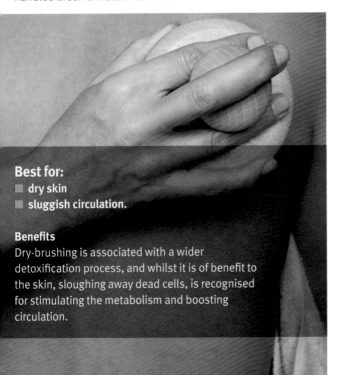

Best for:
- dry skin
- sluggish circulation.

Benefits

Dry-brushing is associated with a wider detoxification process, and whilst it is of benefit to the skin, sloughing away dead cells, is recognised for stimulating the metabolism and boosting circulation.

• KEY POINT

The natural pattern of exfoliation covers the whole body including the buttocks and around the breast area. Always ensure your client has been specifically informed of this. Check and gain their permission to treat these areas.

A word about circadian rhythms

Circadian rhythms are your body's natural hormone fluctuations throughout the day which act to help you wake up in the morning, and feel sleepy at night. Due to its metabolism boosting properties, dry-brushing should be performed to fit with the body's natural circadian rhythms. During the morning 'wake up' hormones such as cortisol are at their peak, and can be further stimulated by the invigorating process of dry-brushing. This will provide a metabolic advantage for the rest of the day. In the evening, however, this process should be avoided, as it may artificially stimulate these hormones and cause sleep disturbances.

Technique

1) Start with the client lying on their front. Brush the lower body starting with firm sweeps to the right foot and right sole, then in long sweeping movements up the right calf followed by the exterior and then interior of the thigh in long sweeps towards the nearest lymph nodes and in the direction of the heart.
2) Continue on the left leg.
3) Brush the buttocks if client has indicated they are comfortable with this area in short firm sweeps moving from the right to left side of the body.
4) Use extra strokes on areas of the upper thigh and buttocks where cellulite can be seen.
5) Proceed to upper body brushing right arm and then left in long sweeps from hand to armpit.
6) Brush upper back towards heart and then lower back in long sweeping strokes.

7) Turn client and repeat body brushing steps 1 to 2 on front of legs.

8) Brush abdomen in light clockwise motions to follow the natural path of digestion.

9) Having obtained the clients consent, brush from the sternum through and around the breasts using small strokes, towards the heart.

10) Alternatively lay the client on their back and begin by brushing the left foot then underneath the left leg. Repeat on the right. Sit the client up and brush the whole back. Gently lay the client back down and brush each arm using upward strikes towards the heart followed by the chest abdomen and front of legs as previously described.

11) Use a smaller brush to gently brush the face in circular motion from forehead to chin.

12) The skin should show an erythema.

13) If the client is to receive further spa treatments they should shower at this stage.

• KEY POINT

Dry-brushing is a technique which clients can be encouraged to continue in their own homes, as the brushes used are easy to come by and inexpensive. Ideally dry-brushing should be carried out every morning before showering for maximum stimulation to the metabolism, with long strokes always towards the heart.

A loofah is a actually a dried variety of fruit, and its firm texture makes it ideal for exfoliating. Loofahs can be used alone or in conjunction with a body scrub. Due to their open texture they can become lodged with skin cells and should always be thoroughly cleansed and dried after use. Therefore they are better for home use

A word about exfoliation equipment

After use exfoliation tools such as loofahs and dry-brushes will be lodged with dry dead skin cells, which are usually too small to see. These can provide breeding grounds for bacteria, so it is very important that any loofah, brush, or other tool is thoroughly cleansed after every use.

To sanitise loofahs and body brushes, submerge them in boiling water briefly, spray them with alcohol sanitiser, scrub them with a clean cloth and then submerge them again in hot water. Then leave them to dry in a warm airy place.

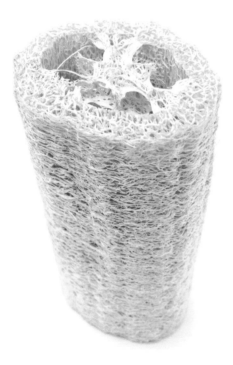

Endpoints

By the end of this topic, you should understand:

- different manual exfoliation methods using equipment such as a dry-brush and loofah
- the potential impact of these methods on natural bodily cycles
- a full technique for exfoliating using a dry-brush or loofah
- caring for exfoliation equipment and keeping it clean.

Topic 5: Scrubs

There are a wide variety of scrubs and exfoliating products available. All involve slightly different levels of abrasiveness and so are suitable for different skin types.

Scrubs generally consist of three major ingredients:

Exfoliant

This is the part of the scrub which gives it texture and sloughs away skin cells. Traditional ingredients include salt, silica sand, rice bran, jojoba beads, apricot kernels, and coffee grains. Biodegradable exfoliants are much preferred as they dissolve upon use unlike synthetic granules.

Oil/moisturiser

This binds the oil exfoliant and also adds a moisturising element to the skin. The best tend to be nut oils such as sweet almond, but other oils such as olive oil are sometimes used. A suspension moisturiser can also take the place of oil.

Perfume/active ingredient

This either fragrances the blend, has some additional aromatherapy or therapeutic property, or both. Examples might include caffeine which is now thought to reduce cellulite, or essential oils such as juniper, black pepper or lemongrass.

Salt glow treatment

Salt glow treatments are an increasingly popular way to team the exfoliating properties of salt with its detoxifying qualities. The treatment is a body scrub using sea salt and aromatic oils. Two to four pounds of fine kiln salt is used and due to the sodium content, moisture and toxins are drawn out the of skin, whilst vasodilatation and desquamation are increased.

• KEY POINT

In general, lighter exfoliants are suitable for younger, more sensitive, and dry skins, whilst stronger scrubs work best on older, and oily skins.

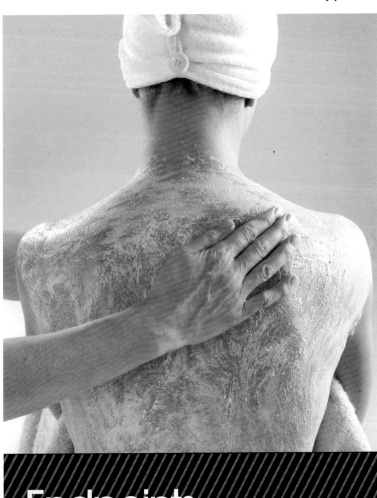

Endpoints

By the end of this topic, you should understand:

- ■ the composition of an exfoliation scrub
- ■ different blends and ingredients
- ■ salt glow treatments and their composition.

TOPIC 6: AFTER CARE

Exfoliation treatments are usually followed by other treatments such as massage, depilation or the application of creams or tanning solutions. Whilst each of these procedures will have its own aftercare rituals, it should be remembered that exfoliation alone will call for specific care to be taken.

Moisturising

After exfoliation, moisturising is the vital next step. This is also important if you are proceeding to another treatment such as false tan, but should not be undertaken prior to waxing.

Exfoliation stimulates sebum production, and if moisturising does not take place can make oily skin produce excess sebum. Conversely, dry skins can become tight and uncomfortable if they are left un-moisturised after exfoliation.

Hydration

As with massage, exfoliation works with the lymphatic system to speed up detoxification in the body. Detoxification relies heavily on adequate water to help flush away substances, and giving the lymph a boost without hydration support will put the body under strain. Without plenty of water, the client could suffer from headaches, aching joints and minor spots as toxins are released without being properly excreted. In the longer term this is still beneficial for the client, but in the short term they should be advised as to how to avoid these symptoms.

A litre or more of (preferably) mineral water should be consumed during the hours following treatment, but remember that excessive water (over a litre an hour continuously) is very dangerous. Mineral water is free from minor toxins such as chlorine found in tap water, which will greater aid its detoxification benefits.

Sun exposure/tanning beds

Sun-tanning shouldn't take place immediately after exfoliation, and clients should be discouraged from sun-bathing for 48 hours after a treatment as skin is more sensitive to heat. In the longer term good exfoliation will mean the resulting tan is likely

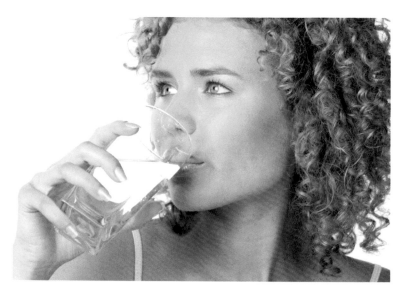

to be deeper and more long-lived. Exfoliation is also encouraged each day to slough off dead skin cells and maintain a smooth even tan.

Additionally, exfoliation is highly recommended immediately prior to false tanning application as it renders the skin smooth prior to application of the product.

Endpoints

By the end of this topic, you should understand:

■ the need for comprehensive aftercare advice following exfoliation.

04

Tanning

Tanning through false tanning products or UV facilities is an increasingly popular way to add a healthy glow to skin. Many beauty therapy outlets now provide false tanning or have access to UV sun-beds or booths as part of their wider treatment programme.

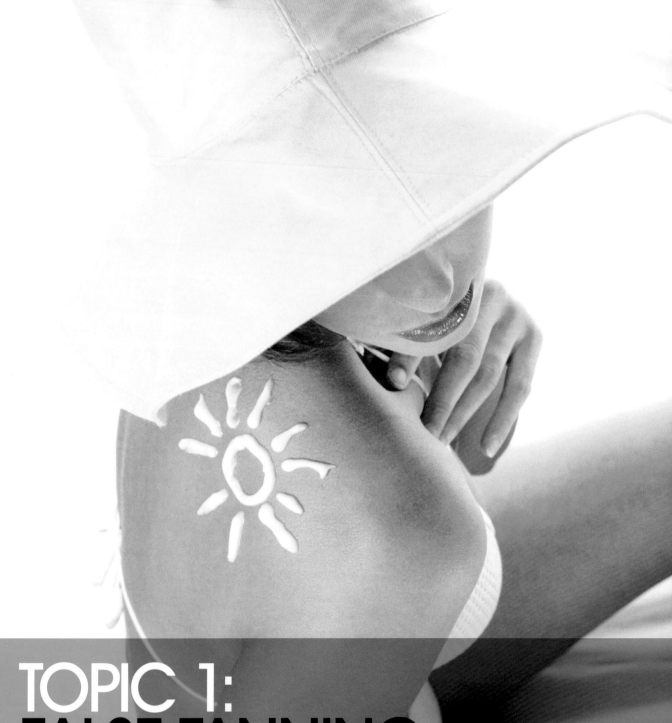

TOPIC 1:
FALSE TANNING

False tans or False tan products are a useful way of getting a healthy glow without exposing the body to the damage of UV light. Sunlight is one of the major factors in premature ageing of the skin, and false tanning products can be used to give a natural look without risk to skin health.

CHECKLIST
Advantages or false tanning
- No damage from harmful UV rays, and subsequent premature ageing
- No need for exposure to UV light
- Tanning is possible all year round
- False tanning can prolong an existing tan
- False tanning products can be applied to specific areas only – e.g. face
- Psychological well-being of healthy glow can be achieved easily
- False tanning products can be used to even out pigmentation disorders.

The science of false tanning

As we have seen in the last chapter, the skin is comprised of several different layers. False tanning products work in the uppermost part of the epidermis – the strateum corneum, where cells have died and become keratinised to form the hard-wearing surface of the skin. Sugars in self or 'fake' tanning products interact with these dead cells to create a colour change.

As the skin is constantly renewing itself, the colour change will last only as long as the dead cells take to slough off and be reformed – around five to seven days with a quality product, professional application and good aftercare.

● DID YOU KNOW?

False tanning products have been around for many years, but it is only relatively recently that the technology has developed to allow them to work with the skin's natural pigmentation. For this reason client's need not fear an 'orange' cast to their skin which was associated with heavy use of old-fashioned false tanning products.

Contraindications

False tanning products are generally very safe and suitable for a wide variety of skin types, including those with pigmentation disorders. They work by using the skin's own natural colouration and

● KEY POINT

False tanning is often preferable for very pale skins, that cannot achieve a natural tan.

rarely cause a reaction. It is, however, imperative that proper precautions such as patch tests are adhered to in case of allergic reaction.

The following are contraindications for false tanning.

CONGENITAL

Congenital means skin conditions which are an ongoing complaint – something which the client is likely to have lived with for a long time. Often these type of skin problems flare up and are worsened by stress, so can be aided by relaxing beauty treatments.

Psoriasis

This is a condition caused by excess skin production, and is thought to be due to an overactive immune system. Some clients do find that light exfoliation with a very mild scrub such as oatmeal can be beneficial, but others find it makes the condition worse. Active psoriasis should be contraindicated to exfoliation.

Blocked sweat glands

These are less common in cold countries as they tend to occur from a combination of excess sweating and dead skin cells. The resulting condition is known as 'prickly heat' and is an uncomfortable rash. Exfoliation should not be undertaken in the event of this condition.

Eczema

Like psoriasis, this is now thought to be due to an overactive immune system and causes sore inflamed skin. Active eczema should be contraindicated to exfoliation.

Dermatitis

This is a blanket term used to refer to any inflammation of the skin. Do not exfoliate skin which is sore, cracked or inflamed.

Inflamed varicose veins

Whilst pronounced varicose veins can often be a good candidate for gentle stimulation by exfoliation, you should not exfoliate directly over sore or inflamed veins. Check with your client if you are unsure.

INFESTATIONS

Infestations refer to conditions where a parasite is living in or on the host – in this case the infected human. This means creatures sometimes too small to be seen with the human eye are living in or under the skin. Whilst you may not be able to see the parasite itself, however, you will be able to see physical signs (rash, inflamed skin) or symptoms (itching) of the infestation.

Scabies

Scabies is an infestation of microscopic mites which burrow under the skin, causing a raised itchy rash all over the body. Scabies is very infectious and no attempt should be made to treat a patient suffering from this condition. Additionally, any area in which an infected person has been in contact should be thoroughly cleansed.

Lice

A body lice infestation is extremely rare on spa users, as lice are the result of very unsanitary body care, and it is highly unlikely that you will encounter this condition as a therapist. Head lice, however are reasonably common, particularly amongst those who have contact with children. These can be identified by small white eggs in the hair and itching. It is easily treated by over-the-counter remedies.

Head lice are infectious, but only if infected hair is brought into direct contact with another scalp. If you notice an infection, tactfully alert the client and ensure any areas in which their head has been in contact has been treated. You may also consider treating your own hair if there is a risk you have been contaminated.

VIRAL

Viral infections enter the cells of the body, and burrow into the nucleus, where they can hijack the body's own mechanisms to make new versions of themselves. Even after an infection has taken hold and been overcome by the immune system, the virus still lies hidden in the nucleus. They then appear to be able to sense when the body is under stress (and therefore in weakened immunity) and use this time to reproduce and re-infect.

As viruses are long-lived in this way, and can reoccur throughout a lifetime, they are particularly unpleasant conditions to contract, and great care should be taken to avoid contamination and infection.

Warts

Warts are a viral infection, which the body usually rids itself of after a lengthy period of time. They are infectious, and you should avoid treating areas of the body with warts.

Herpes Simplex

Otherwise known as cold-sores, herpes is extremely common and it is estimated 60% of people carry the virus. As long as you are not treating the facial area, treatments can be carried out on a client with cold sores, but you should take extra hygiene precautions and avoid touching your own face during treatment.

FUNGAL

Fungal infections are usually localised to one part of the body, with the feet being particularly vulnerable. They can be treated and cleared up permanently, but are infectious and care should be taken to avoid contamination.

Fungal problems usually occur when an imbalance of conditions such as acidity or yeast allow fungus to grow out of control, overwhelming the body's natural mechanisms of restoring normal conditions.

BACTERIAL

This is a general term, but usually applies to an infection of the feet. It is characterised by flaky white skin around the toes, scaly, flaking toenails, yellowing toenails or distortions of the toenails as the bacteria raises them from the toes. Generally speaking it is possible to treat clients with foot disorders as long as a pair of socks are worn.

Ringworm

Ringworm is a fungal infection which grows into a raised red ring. It can also form other shapes, but is generally characterised by a line of raised skin. It is infectious, and contact should be avoided until the condition has been treated by a medical professional.

SKIN INJURY

Any kind of injury from a small scratch or bruise to a more serious abrasion should not be exfoliated, or be subject to treatment from other creams or treatments such as fake tan.

Additionally the following conditions would indicate a client would not be suitable for false tan application.

- **Broken or damaged skin.** Never apply false tan to broken, cut, or damaged skin. It is, however, possible to carefully work around an isolated area of injury.
- **Sunburn.** False tan should not be applied to skin which has been burnt in the sun.
- **Peeling/flaking skin.** This might be due to sunburn, or other skin conditions. Skin which is flaking from the body even after exfoliation will make it impossible to apply and even tan. The product will become lodged in the dry skin and give a mottled effect.
- **Dermatitis.** This refers to many different skin disorders including eczema and psoriasis, but the result is skin which is broken, open, inflamed, itching, and otherwise untreatable. If in doubt suggest a client consult their doctor. It is, however, often possible to carefully treat around small patches of dermatological disorders.

• KEY POINT

You are legally liable for any allergic reaction resulting from a treatment which you administer, and so patch tests should be rigorously adhered to. If a client has already been tested you must insist they sign the consultation form to ensure you are not liable if they have misinformed you and/ or react to a product.

PATCH TEST

It is vital to carry out a patch test to ensure a client doesn't have an allergy to the tanning product being used. Ideally this should be carried out even if a client has previously had a false tan treatment with a different brand to the one you are using.

1) Take a small amount of the product you are using on a spatula.
2) Apply a dab to the client's inner wrist or the crook of their elbow.
3) The product needs to remain unwashed in place for 24 hours.
4) Following this test the client should report if any adverse reaction has taken place, such as reddening of the skin, inflammation or itching.

Endpoints

By the end of this topic, you should understand:

- the advantages to false tanning over UV tanning
- science behind how false tanning products work
- contraindications which could prevent treatment
- how to carry out a patch test and the importance of doing so.

TOPIC 2:
PREPARATION FOR FALSE TANNING

As a skin preparation false tanning products will work much more effectively and last longer with correct preparation of the skin. Where possible you should inform the client of the best prior conditions for applying false tan professionally so they can enjoy the greatest benefits.

PREPARATION

The client's skin needs to be very clean before a treatment, and ideally have been professionally exfoliated (see Chapter 3: Exfoliation). If you have the facilities the client can shower immediately before the tan application for best results.

False tan is a form of dye, and can stain fabrics so for this reason extreme caution should be taken with the product when applying it for treatment.

Hair removal

As the client is advised not to shave or wax for several days after product application, it is advisable to encourage hair removal shortly before treatment. If the client waxes then two to three days should be left between the hair removal and false tan application. Shaving can take place shortly before.

Client dress

The client should be allowed to disrobe with the usual professional care for modesty, and disposable underwear provided. All jewellery apart from the wedding band should be removed.

Preparing the area

Extra care should be taken in protecting the treatment couch with plastic wrap and paper towels as appropriate. You should also wear suitable protective clothing and plastic or latex gloves.

Exfoliation

For effective coverage and longevity false tan should be allowed to penetrate the skins layers evenly and effectively. Exfoliation removes dead skins cells and gives the false tan the best base for working on the skin.

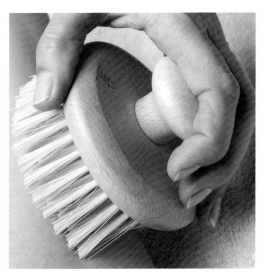

Moisturise

A natural tan will tend to settle more deeply on more oil-rich areas of the body such as the stomach and shoulders. In contrast false tan will be soaked up proportionally more by dryer areas of skin such as elbows, knees and heels.

This makes it vitally important that moisturiser is properly applied to reverse the tendency of false tan to favour spots where the sun would not naturally tan so deeply, and will ensure your client emerges with a natural-looking tan.

APPLYING MOISTURISER FOR OPTIMAL FALSE TANNING

Start with the heels. You should not apply false tan to this area, so apply a thick layer of moisturiser to where the tan line should end to prevent staining.

Apply moisturiser thickly to elbows and knees.

Moisturise shins well, particularly if they are dry. If there is scaly skin in this area, moisturise heavily, wipe off with a clean towel to sweep away excess skin, and reapply a thinner layer.

Continue with the rest of the body.

If excess moisturiser remains on elbows and knees by the time the body has been moisturised, remove it with paper towels.

Always follow manufacturer's instructions as they vary greatly form product to product.

Endpoints
By the end of this topic, you should understand:

- the various factors which are optimal for the application of False tan
- application of moisturiser in varying thicknesses to different parts of the body prior to false tan application.

TOPIC 3:
TANNING PRODUCTS

There are a variety of different tanning products on the market and as a professional price will be a consideration as well as results. Therapists often report, however, that more expensive products are easier to apply and are used in smaller amounts so may be more cost effective with careful application.

APPLICATIONS OF FALSE TANNING PRODUCT

False tanning products come in different application types, from smooth creams to light mousses or spray-on. The type you use will usually depend on the preference of the salon in which you work.

1) Creams and lotions

Creams and lotions are usually dark coloured already, which helps in the application, as streaking can be corrected immediately. They do, however, take practice to apply in even strokes

● KEY POINT

Although different applications and varieties of false tanning products exist, the ingredients used are the same. It is only the style of application which differs.

which ensure an even-looking false tan. Some products contain a darker colour to guide the therapist as to where the product has been applied and to help avoid gaps and streaking.

2) Mousses

Mousses have a light aerated texture, which means they are not absorbed as quickly as creams, which can make for better tanning application. Mousses are often favoured for home application, where they can make tanning hard-to-reach parts of the body easier.

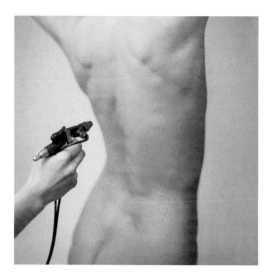

3) Sprays

Spray tans of the hand-held kind are widely used in beauty salons. Their advantage is that they apply evenly and dry quickly, which is helpful if applying in a home environment. A beauty therapist, however, will be able to work a cream, or lotion into a perfect even coverage. Spray tanning booths, however, are now a popular way to enjoy a professionally applied false tan.

4) Airbrushing/spray tan

This is fake tan which is professionally applied by hand with an airbrushing device. They allow the client to be finely misted with product in a standing position, meaning full-body application in a matter of minutes and very fast drying times. Training is needed to use the equipment, but airbrushed tan is fast to apply, can give even coverage, and can also be built up at the request of the client to even out paler areas and give a uniform colour.

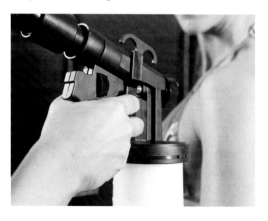

5) Automated booths

As the name suggests these automated booths give an all-over even coverage of spray tan in a private booth. The automated nature allow for less margin for error than a hand-applied airbrush tan, but the application is the same for every client and does not compensate for paler areas. A major advantage is the modesty factor, as clients may enter the booth privately once they are undressed.

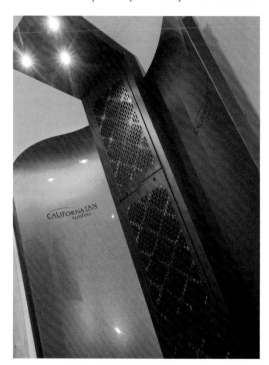

ON THE LABEL

False tanning products work with some basic scientific ingredients which enact a change in the colour of the skin. Whilst these may look complex the core chemicals used are basically the same, with only slight differences between them.

Dihydroxy acetone (DHA)

A professional tan will usually have DHA on the label. This is the active ingredient which reacts just below the skin surface to create a browning effect. Unlike stains or pigments it is the effect of enzymes in the skin and is similar to the reaction found when foods brown. For this reason it is the body's own colouration being used, and the result is a natural colour well suited to the individual.

Tyrosine

Tyrosine is a 'tan-accelerator' which can be used in pill form or in lotions to increase the formation of melanin – the body's natural sun-tan pigment. There is still some debate as to whether this ingredient is effective.

Erythrulose

Similarly to DHA, erythrulose produces a browning effect on the skin by reacting with naturally occurring proteins. Erythrulose tans develop more slowly and are lighter than DHA based tans, and also fade more quickly. The colouration is also described by some as a redder hue than the DHA tan, fading can be blotchy and it is a more expensive ingredient, so DHA is usually used in professional products for preference.

In the case of an allergy to a DHA based product, however erythrulose can be a useful substitute. As usual, a patch test should be carried out 24 hours in advance of application.

APPLYING A LOTION-BASED TAN

- Always read the manufacturer's instructions, as products vary.
- Monitor skin reaction as you apply the product – look out for any reddening or signs of discomfort.
- Wipe over any areas of dry skin with damp cotton wool pads after application to ensure they do not absorb too much of the product.
- Apply the product smoothly and fill in any streaks. There should be no visible lines.
- For facial application, mix the product with 50% moisturiser to give a subtler look.

Endpoints

By the end of this topic, you should understand:

- different application formulations of false tan, such as creams, sprays and mousses
- ingredients of false tan products and how they differ in effect
- basic application techniques for a lotion-based false tan product.

TOPIC 4: PIGMENTATION DISORDERS

False tanning treatments can be a very effective way to lessen the appearance of pigmentation disorders and even out skin tone. As they can be applied to small areas a pigmented patch of skin can be carefully coloured to reduce contrasting colouration patches.

There are several types of pigmentation disorder, ranging from those which stain patches of the skin, to those which interfere with natural melanin giving a mottled appearance.

This is a rare condition in which the cells in the skin responsible for pigment die or become unable to function. It is not well understood, and can be very distressing for the individual concerned. The appearance is particularly pronounced on dark-skin.

False tan can be used to even out patches of unpigmented skin, making them darker. It is not possible to restore skin to a pigmented appearance, but considerable improvements can be made. It is most effective on larger patches of skin. Clients seeking this treatment should consult their doctor prior to undertaking false tanning, as specialist tanning products may be required.

This is a condition whereby the natural pigmentation of the skin does not work, leaving an individual with all over very white skin. False tan can work well on this condition, but it doesn't last as long as with ordinary pigmented skin.

1) Chloasma (melasma)
This is a hyper pigmentation of the skin, resulting in dark patches similar in appearance to liver spots. It particularly affects pregnant women, and certain ethnic groups are also disproportionately affected. It is thought to be hormone-related and will usually fade naturally. False tan can help

disguise this pigmentation by tanning the skin surrounding the darker patches and evening out skin tone.

2) Ephilides
This is another term for freckles. Freckles are usually exacerbated by UV exposure. The resulting pigmentation can be evened out slightly by false tanning products.

3) Port wine stain
This is a heavy red pigmentation of the skin caused by deep capillary dilation. There is no reason not to false tan skin stained in this manner, but the product will not have any effect on pigmented areas. If a client is undergoing laser treatment for port wine stain, false tanning should be avoided.

Leucoderma
Like vitiligo, this is a pigment disorder which causes white spots and patches on the skin. False tan can help even out skin tone if applied in greater quantities to paler areas.

Naevae
Otherwise known as a birth mark. If pigmented this may occur on any part of the body and is often found on the neck and face being sometimes associated with strong hair growth. These vary in size from pinhead to several centimetres and in rare cases may be extremely large. Pigmentation

varies from light brown to black. Strawberry naevae (pink or red birth marks) often affect babies, eventually disappearing after a few years.

Moles (papilloma)

A common occurrence on the face and body and present in several different forms varying in size, colour and vascular appearance. Flat moles are called sessile whilst those raised above the surface or attached by a stalk are pedunculated.

URITICARA/ALLERGIC REACTIONS

Always consult with a client who has a pigment disorder as to the nature of the problem. More importantly, never assume that a false tanning client with red patches of skin is suffering from a disorder of pigmentation rather than something which could be a contraindication.

Uriticara is an allergic reaction which causes inflamed raised red patches of the skin. False tan should not be applied to clients suffering with uriticara, or any other allergic reaction as it can worsen symptoms.

• KEY POINT

If you are unsure as to whether a client has a pigmentation disorder you need to find out before you treat them. But ensure you approach the topic in a tactful and polite manner.

Endpoints

By the end of this topic, you should understand:

- the various pigmentation disorders possible on the skin
- effect of false tanning product on these disorders
- that not all pigmentation disorders will be modified by false tan, and the effect is not a cure for the condition
- the importance of not confusing a more serious skin contraindication with a pigmentation disorder.

TOPIC 5: AFTERCARE

Keeping the false tan looking its best and lasting as long as possible is the goal of a professional application. Good exfoliation and professional application with judicious application of moisturiser will go a long way to achieving this end. However, false tanning aftercare should be impressed on the client for best results.

PREVENTING FADING

As we have seen earlier in this chapter, false tans work in the strateum corneum of the epidermis. This means as the skin sheds the tan will fade. For this reason any process which accelerates the shedding of the skin will hasten the fading of the tan.

In the first twelve hours after application

The following precautions/advice should be given for activities immediately after false tanning application.

Loose fitting clothing

The client should avoid wearing tight clothing which can rub away the tan, resulting both in decreased effectiveness of the product and also staining to clothes. Very tight clothes combined with chafing and sweating could cause white patches on the skin where the product has been entirely rubbed away.

Bathing/showering

For a period immediately after application clients should not bath or shower. This is because the false tan is still being absorbed into the skin, and washing it away will lessen the amount which soaks into the epidermis and subsequently causes long-lasting colouration. The time period for this will be specified by the particular product you are using, but is usually around eight hours.

Beauty products
The client should also avoid using any products on top of the false tan during this period such as moisturiser, exfoliating scrubs, or perfume.

Beauty treatments
Treatments such as massage, waxing and body masks can all lead to premature fading of the false tan, and treatments might also react adversely with the product.

Perspiration
Perspiring (sweating) can speed up the production of skin cells, but more importantly the sweat can also force the tanning product back out of the pores.

For this reason clients should be properly cautioned to avoid activities where they are likely to perspire heavily for twelve hours after the product application. These would include:

- **Heavy aerobic exercise such as running**
- **Saunas and steam rooms**
- **Hot or bikram yoga**
- **Sunbed**
- **Hot baths.**

For the entire five-to-seven-day period after treatment
During the period following the first twelve hours the client can increase the longevity of their false tan.

• KEY POINT

For false tan which has been applied to the face, the client should sip hot drinks through a straw for the first twelve hours or so, as hot drinks can strip false tan from around the mouth.

Moisturising
Locking in the skin's moisture is key to preventing the upper most cells drying out and flaking away. Clients should be encouraged to moisturise regularly and especially after showering, as warm water evaporating from the skin will lose moisture.

Exfoliation
Whilst exfoliation is usually recommended for healthy skin, for the purposes of false tanning perseveration it should be avoided for at least five days. Harsh scrubs, body brushing, and even rough towels can all hasten the fading of a false tan. Shaving will have the same effect.

Other things to avoid
- **Products containing alpha hydroxyl acids (AHAs). These are found in anti-ageing skin products and can strip false tan.**
- **Chlorinated swimming pools can fade tan colour.**

Sun exposure
Most clients are aware that exposure to sun can result in damage to skin, but with the application of a false tan it is sometimes easy to forget that the colour does not confer the same protection as a sun-induced tan. Remind your clients to use a good quality sun block, and emphasise that a false tan will not protect their skin from UV damage.

Endpoints
By the end of this topic, you should understand:

- the need for aftercare to maximise false tan treatment.
- differences in aftercare needed at different times following treatment.

TOPIC 6: UV TANNING

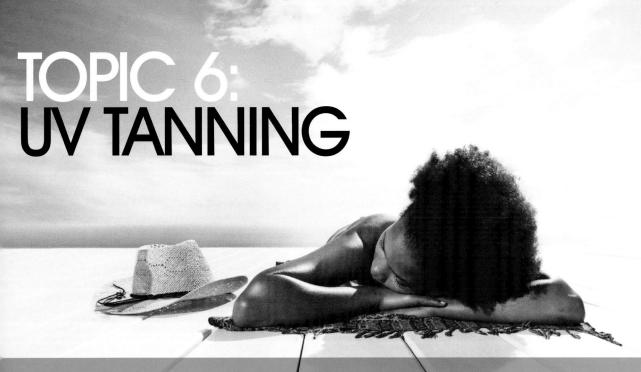

Tanning using UV equipment allows clients to gain a natural long-lasting tan all year round. UV light can also have benefits for medical conditions such as acne. There is a certain degree of controversy surrounding UV tanning, and as a therapist you should be well-informed as to potential side effects from misuse as well as benefits.

THE ELECTROMAGNETIC SPECTRUM

The electromagnetic spectrum refers to the entire range of rays from the sun, spanning radiowaves at one end of the scale right the way through the visible light of colours we can see to so-called 'ultra violet' rays. These are transmitted as energy which can affect the pigmentation of the skin, and comprise UVA, UVB, and UVC rays.

You can read in more detail about the electromagnetic spectrum and different types of light in Chapter 10.

UVA

UVA refers to 'Ultra Violet Light' and are the rays responsible for skin-ageing. They penetrate deep into the dermis, damaging the collagen support which gives skin youthful plumpness. UVA rays from tanning equipment work by stimulating melanin in skin which is already tanned. For this reason it is not as long lasting as a tan gained through sun exposure.

UVB

These are the rays which are responsible for sunburn, and for this reason tanning equipment tends to use mainly UVA rays with minute amounts of UVB. This allows the UVA to penetrate the dermis without burning the skin, and as UVA does not stimulate the epidermis to thicken and protect itself, more UVA can reach the dermis using artificial tanning equipment.

UVC

These are part of the ultra violet spectrum, but are absorbed by the atmosphere before they reach the earth. They are lethal to living things.

Tanning – the production of melanin

The production of melanin or melanogenesis is the reason skin acquires the darkened colouration known as tanning.

1) UV rays are absorbed by the skin, where it enters the basal layers of the epidermis.

2) Here they stimulate an enzyme called tyrosinase which is present in melonocytes – pigment forming cells.

3) The enzyme works to transform a colourless amino acid into the dark coloured melanin.

4) Melanin migrates upwards towards the surface of the skin, giving the skin a tanned appearance.

BENEFITS OF UV EXPOSURE

Although exposure to UV light is associated with skin damage, short controlled exposure is associated with benefits. These include:

Healthy appearance

Tanned skin is associated with good health, and for most clients the main reason for frequenting a UV tanning facility will be for beauty benefits. Tanning can also even out skin tone and give a golden glow.

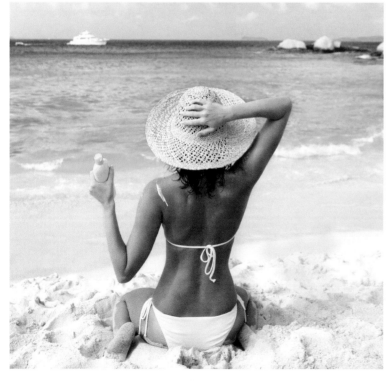

Warming /relaxing the skin

The heat benefits of being under UV light are to relax the muscles and bring blood supply to the skin surface. This effect is covered in more detail in Chapter 5: Heat treatments.

Synthesis of vitamin D

The skin is one of the body's main sources of vitamin D, which it synthesises from sunlight. In cooler climates such as the UK there is now widespread evidence to show many people are deficient in vitamin D, especially during the winter months.

Acne/pimple control

UV light acts as a strong antibacterial agent, and is often recommended by GPs for clients suffering from acne. The treatment will often lessen the condition, destroying bacteria in and on the skin.

Skin diseases

Many clients use sunbeds to treat long-term skin conditions. Common reasons for this include eczema and psoriasis which can benefit from UV exposure.

Seasonal Affective Disorder - SAD

Seasonally specific bouts of depression have now been proven in some cases to be light dependent. This means that in the absence of sunlight the patient suffers from low mood and even depression. Treatment for this can take the form of a specialised light box, but UV light is also effective.

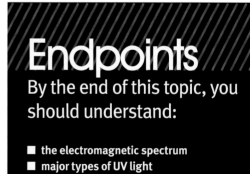

Endpoints

By the end of this topic, you should understand:

- the electromagnetic spectrum
- major types of UV light
- advantages of UV treatment.

TOPIC 7:
PRIOR TO TREATMENT

UV tanning should always be treated with utmost caution and the proper preparations made. These include both informing the client as to all aspects of the treatment as well as modifying their exposure time in accordance to their skin type.

The client should ideally shower immediately before treatment, and a professional exfoliation treatment is preferable for best results. All jewellery should be removed, and no heavily perfumed products should be used prior.

Patch test

As with false tanning treatments, a patch test is necessary both for the client's safety and your legal protection.

1) Have the client lie face down in the tanning equipment with their back exposed.
2) Cut a small hole from a large piece of salon paper-towel and place it over the exposed skin, leaving a small portion bare to the UV rays.
3) Expose the client to UV for one minute.
4) Check the reaction of the skin immediately for redness or undesirable pigmentation.
5) Check again after a 24 hour period adverse reactions.

Tanning products

Products such as tanning accelerators can be used in conjunction with UV equipment. Always follow the manufacturer's guidelines. Any problems experienced with such products should be reported immediately to the relevant person in charge.

ASCERTAINING TREATMENT TIME

The patch test can also be used to ascertain correct treatment times, however the main information used in this process should be the manufacturer's guidelines. Tanning equipment varies considerably, and depending on the power

• KEY POINT

UV is a very powerful tool, and therapists should be very aware of their duty of care to the client. Usage on sensitive skins can result in painful damage, long-lasting injury to the skin or even permanent pigmentation.

and age of the machinery can make a significant difference to exposure times recommended.

Using timers

Timers on UV equipment are manufactured according to the specifications of maximum exposure, and should never be overridden.

SKIN TYPES

The beauty industry usually designates six skin types according to how easily the epidermis develops pigmentation on sun exposure. The first four skin types are usually Caucasian (white) skinned, with types five and six relating to brown or black skin.

Type I. Always burns easily, and can even blister under limited sun exposure. Due to the severity of reaction to the sun, skin then peels meaning a tan almost never develops. Usual features are blue eyes, fair hair and very light skin.

Type II. Usually burns easily and peels, although can develop a light tan. Red or blonde hair, blue or hazel eyes and fair skin.

Type III. Unprotected skin will burn quite quickly, but a golden tan can develop. This is the average Caucasian skin tone.

Type IV. Burning can occur but tanning is more usual and will develop quickly to a dark colour. This type is usually people of Oriental, Hispanic, or Mediterranean descent. Often shows Immediate Pigment Darkening reaction (IPD) where exposed skin will instantly pigment.

Type V. Rarely burns, always tans, and always pigments immediately (IPD). Unexposed skin is brown and darkens further under UV.

Type VI. Tans rapidly and never burns. IPD reaction always evident. Persons with very dark (black) skin, such as those of African or Aboriginal heritage.

MED

MED stands for Minimal Erythema Dosage, and relates to the amount of exposure needed to turn the skin a barely discernable shade of pink. This is the maximum desirable exposure required to cause a gradual tanning of the skin with minimal UV damage.

PREPARATION CHECKLIST

- Client should ideally shower before treatment.
- Perfumed preparations and jewellery should be removed apart from wedding band.
- Goggles or similar eye coverings are provided, and client is advised on the importance of their use.
- UV patch test has been carried out. Timer has been checked and set.

CONTRAINDICATIONS

UV tanning is not suitable for everyone, and particular care should be taken to ascertain that a client is not suffering from a condition which would make it dangerous for them to use tanning equipment.

- Pregnancy
- Cardio vascular conditions (thrombosis, phlebitis, hypertension, hypotension, heart conditions)
- Any condition already being treated by a GP or dermatologist
- Medical oedema (water retention)
- Nervous/psychotic conditions
- Fever

- Contagious or infectious diseases
- Under the influence of recreational drugs or alcohol
- Diarrhoea and vomiting
- Skin cancer
- Photosensitive skins
- Urticaria
- Medication which causes the skin to become photosensitive, e.g. antibiotics, some blood pressure medication, tranquillisers, malaria treatment if they are planning on travelling to an at risk area and are taking treatment in advance, or have just returned.
- After any form of heat treatment
- After waxing
- After electrolysis
- Excessive moles (more than 100)
- Contact lenses (unless removed)
- Epilepsy
- Recent operations
- Diabetes
- Asthma
- Bells palsy
- Trapped/pinched nerve
- Inflamed nerve
- Acute rheumatism
- Pigmentation disorders such as vitiligo or albinism
- Hypersensitive skins
- Highly vascular skins
- Undiagnosed lumps and bumps
- Scar tissues (two years for major operation and six months for a small scar)
- Sunburn
- Areas of undiagnosed pain
- Any metal pins or plates
- After a heavy meal (sunbeds only)
- Recent X-ray (three months)
- Any other contraindications which you suspect could restrict treatment.

GP permission

If you suspect a client has a contraindication, but they maintain they are fit to receive tanning treatment, you must ensure they obtain and supply you with a suitable note from their GP. This note must contain explicit information regarding UV tanning on a sun-bed.

Where GP permission cannot be obtained a

client must sign an informed consent before undergoing treatment. This consent should be available as a standard document in anywhere which supplies UV tanning, and if this form is not available you should inform the relevant personnel. The form should include confirmation that the client is fully aware of the risks of undergoing treatment and is willing to proceed without permission from their GP.

Endpoints

By the end of this topic, you should understand:

- optimal preparation for the skin prior to tanning
- how to perform a patch test for UV
- ascertaining different skin types
- judging treatment times based on individual clients
- possible contraindications which could make tanning inappropriate.

TOPIC 8:
OVEREXPOSURE

UV light can damage the skin, and therapists must be trained in how to avoid over-exposure and to recognise the symptoms. Clients are often tempted to use UV light for longer periods than is advisable, and therapists must be able to counter this desire if necessary.

RECOGNISING OVEREXPOSURE

Over exposure is defined as exposure sufficient to cause erythema, or sun burn. This means that any reddening of the skin is undesirable.

Repeated overexposure is believed to cause eye and skin injury and allergic reactions and increase the risks of developing photo-ageing of the skin, dryness, wrinkling, and (sometimes fatal) skin cancer.

Erythema

Erythema refers to a degree of damage made by UV light. In order for the skin to tan it must have some reaction to UV, but the skill of the therapist is to ensure this is at the minimal possible level to ensure tanning without long-term damage.

● KEY POINT

The risks of over-exposure are extremely severe and therapists should always make it a matter of utmost importance that client's do not overuse UV facilities.

Four stages of erythema

1) First-degree erythema – the skin is a slightly pink shade, and the colouration disappears after 24 hours with no irritation.
2) Second-degree erythema – skin is markedly red with some itching and soreness. Redness lasts for up to three days.
3) Third-degree erythema – very red, hot, burned skin which is very sore and can last up to a week.
4) Fourth-degree erythema – as with third-degree, but with blistering and peeling resulting.

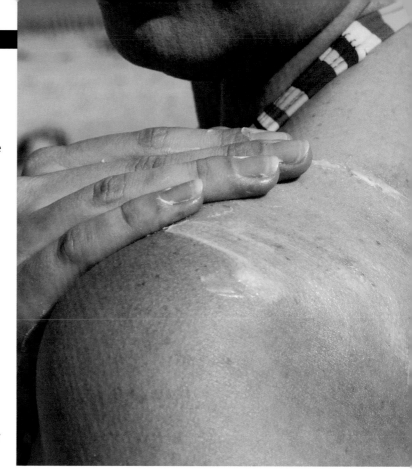

OTHER SIDE EFFECTS

Excess UV light can have additional side effects, which should never occur within the managed dose of light administered therapeutically.

Prickly heat

This is a condition whereby the sweat glands become blocked due to excess sweat being formed. The combination of these two factors then causes the sweat to become trapped in the blocked pore leading irritation and an itchy rash. The condition is not serious and will cure itself within days, but particularly afflicts the very overweight and those prone to excess sweating.

Nausea

In rare cases people can feel nauseous using UV light, mainly due to the heat involved rather than any other factor. If a client complains of nausea they should exit any sun-bed or other equipment immediately. An isolated incident is not necessarily a cause for concern, but if you find more than one client complains of feeling nauseous you should contact the manufacturer of whatever equipment they are using. You may also want to be alert for signs of heat exhaustion (see below).

Thickening of the skin

Excess sunlight can cause thickening of the skin as the epidermis reacts to protect itself. This effect should be minor with exposure to the UVA light found in tanning equipment, as this type of light should avoid the thickening effect.

Small amounts of skin thickening UVB light are used, however, meaning that excessive tanning on UV equipment could cause thickening of the skin. Another possible cause is a malfunction in machinery used, which makes it vitally important this kind of equipment is regularly serviced.

Photo-ageing

The beauty industry believes that properly managed exposure to UV light causes more benefits than harm, and will not make significant damage to skin beyond that which the normal ageing process would generate.

There are some clients, however, who use sun-tanning equipment excessively, possibly combined with exposure to outdoor sunlight, and this can have a very degenerative effect on the skin.

Photo-ageing happens naturally as we get older, and results in thinner skin, lines, wrinkles, and skin pigmentation. UV light can speed up this process, sometimes considerably, and as this is a very undesirable result for a client, excess use of tanning equipment should be guarded against.

Skin cancer

Photo-aged skin undergoes changes and some of this affects the DNA of genes of the skin. Skin cancer is caused by cells in the epidermis multiplying out of control and excess UV light is known to make this effect more likely. In proper conditions there is no reason why a client using tanning equipment should be more at risk from skin cancer, but you should be aware of this very serious risk from overexposure to UV light. Clients should look out for patches of skin which have changed colour or texture, moles which have changed in size, and any unexplained lumps under or in the skin.

Fainting

It is very rare for a client to faint using UV equipment, and all equipment comes with automatic shut-off mechanisms, so a client would not be in danger of overexposing. If a client feels

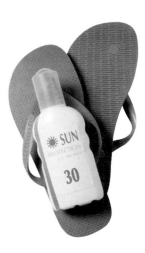

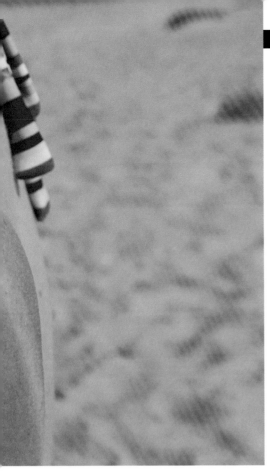

faint, they should immediately cease using any tanning equipment and sit with their head between their legs for a few minutes.

Heat exhaustion

This usually applies to people who have spent considerable periods of time in the sun and heat, and is unlikely to be a concern for those exposed to UV tanning for a few minutes at a time. The main heat exhaustion symptoms include dizziness, nausea (or vomiting), and headache. Skin may be cool and moist, pulse rapid and breathing shallow. Heat exhaustion is more likely in the elderly.

Dehydration

Exposure to UV light will tend to strip some moisture from the body, and clients should be advised to drink plenty of water and use tanning treatment lotions before treatment and moisturisers afterwards to avoid drying of skin. Excess dehydration can also lead to the symptoms of heat exhaustion (see above).

Pigmentation problems

UV light causes skin pigmentation, but sometimes the effect can be to confer uneven pigmentation. These are most commonly in the form of darker

• KEY POINT

Always check up to date procedures on conditions such as heat exhaustion and sun burn with St John's Ambulance, and ensure there is a registered first aider on the premises.

patches of pigmented skin and are the result of overuse of equipment. Clients who report pigmented patches of skin should be dissuaded from continuing to use UV tanning equipment for a time period and to significantly reduce their usage.

Telangiectasia (thread veins)

These are small dilated blood vessels also known as thread veins. They appear near the surface of the skin, particularly in areas of heavy blood flow, such as the upper thighs or backs of the knees. Thread veins can be stimulated by UV light or excess heat.

Skin immunity

Skin has its own immune cells which help counter infection. There is some evidence to suggest that the function of this immune response can be lessened by exposure to UV light. This means the skin is more vulnerable to infection.

Actinic keratosis

This is a build up of crusty scaly skin, usually as a direct result of excessive UV exposure. It is more common on fair skins, and can start as a reddened patch of yellow flaky skin, or a brown build-up similar in appearance to a mole or wart. Since this condition is associated with potential later development of skin cancer it should be treated by a GP, who can remove growths of the condition.

Endpoints

By the end of this topic, you should understand:

- the danger of overexposure on UV tanning equipment
- possible effects and consequences of overexposure
- recognising the signs and symptoms of overexposure.

TOPIC 9: SUNSCREENS

Clients using UV equipment can use sunscreens both to even out tanning, and for skin protection. Where skin is very pale it is imperative that sunscreens are used until a greater resistance to the light is built up.

Many different sunscreens are available for clients to purchase, but there can be a large difference between the effectiveness of the screens.

Sunscreens work by absorbing or blocking UV light, making the skin less vulnerable to sun-damage. They are manufactured in different formulations according to the protective requirement.

Physical sunscreens

Sunscreens act as a total barrier to sunlight. For this reason, clothing, umbrellas and other skin-cover-ups fall into the category of physical sunscreens.

Chemical sunscreens/blocks

Chemical sunscreens are formulated to scatter, absorb, or prevent the penetration of UV rays. They are rated according to the SPF factor system. This means that the numerical protection factor refers to the amount of extra time skin can be exposed to the sun before it will react as if unprotected.

So an SPF factor of 30, for example, would mean that skin which usually burns after ten minutes could be in the sun for 30 times longer – five hours – before this reaction would occur.

• KEY POINT

The best sunscreens will protect from both UVA and UVB light.

• DID YOU KNOW?

Only a few sunscreens work instantly. Most of the chemical sunscreens need around twenty minutes to absorb and work.

They can be categorised as sunblocks and sunscreen:

Sunblock

This is a very high-factor thick barrier which prevents any sunlight making contact with the skin. Zinc oxide is the most commonly used barrier-block. It is formulated as a thick white or coloured cream which is smeared thickly over parts of the body which are particularly vulnerable to burning such as the nose.

Sunscreen

These are the most commonly used sunscreens as they allow light to be absorbed, but at a slower pace than on unprotected skin. Sunscreens usually contain benzophenones for UVA protection, and sometimes cinnamates and salicylates are useful for protecting your skin from UVB rays.

Creams, oils, lotions and milks

Sunscreens come in many different formulations, and for the most part the benefits they confer are identical, but the application method is a matter of preference.

Creams

Creams usually refer to high SPF ratings, as their thicker consistency can give better protection as a partial barrier. They should be rubbed well into the skin to prevent unsightly streaking.

Lotions and milks

This is the most common formulation for sun-bathers, and cover the average SPF range from six to fifty. In general milks are thinner and more easily applied than lotions, but come in lower SPF.

Sun oil

Sun oils are available as tan accelerators, but are not generally recommended for this purpose as they can damage the skin. As a sunscreen, sun oils are usually in a spray bottle, allowing easy application.

Endpoints

By the end of this topic, you should understand:

- the difference between sunblocks and sunscreens
- the chemical properties of certain sunscreens
- SPF factor and what it means for skin protection.

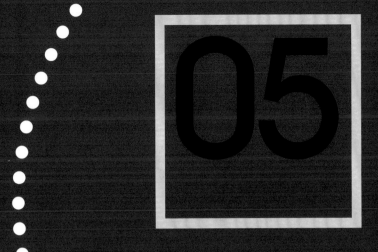

05

Heat treatments

Heated treatments can be a wonderfully soothing way to relax and warm the body prior to treatment, or as a treatment in their own right. There are many benefits to gently pre-heating the body, and whilst facilities such as saunas and steam rooms are commonly associated with larger spas they can in fact be utilised by even the smallest of spa outlets.

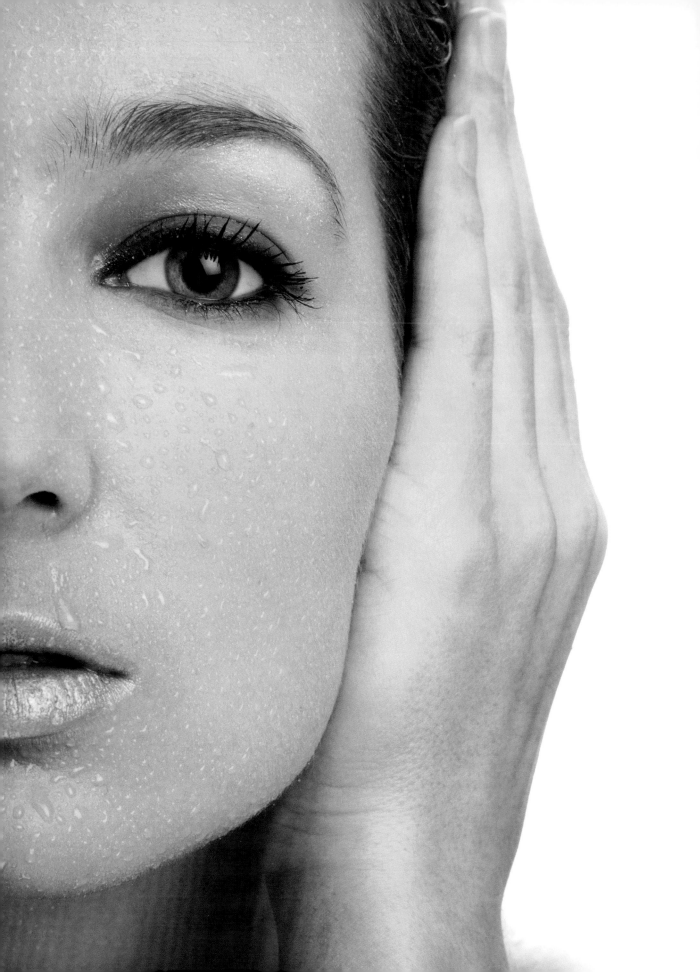

TOPIC 1: BENEFITS OF HEAT TREATMENT

The application of gentle heat to the body comes with a great number of benefits, both for health, appearance of the skin, and responsiveness to later treatments. Most clients find heat treatments to be a relaxing way to prepare for another therapeutic procedure and they are often used in spas for this purpose.

WHAT IS HEAT TREATMENT?

A heat treatment refers to a procedure during which the body is heated for the purposes of health and well-being. The most widely known method of heat treatment is the sauna or steam bath, which has been in existence since Roman times.

BENEFITS OF HEAT THERAPY

1) Relax tense muscles

The main benefit for the body from a therapist's perspective is that a heat treatment will relax tense muscles fibres. This means if a client is undergoing a massage following their heat treatment the muscles will already be some way towards relaxation making work easier for the therapist and more comfortable for the client.

2) Soothe the nerves

Nerve endings are soothed in heated conditions, relaxing the client.

3) Skin colour improved

As the capillaries dilate the skin flushes slightly, bringing a more even colour to the skin. With repeated treatments this effect can help improve the overall texture of the skin.

4) Circulation increased

As the body gets colder blood is brought inwards to keep the internal organs warm. But in heated conditions the opposite effect is reached. Blood is pumped out into the extremities, providing nutrients to the skin, removing waste, and improving tone. Repeated heat treatments are thought to be able to permanently improve poor circulation.

5) Sweat induced

Sweat glands in the skin dilate in order to cool the body. As sweat is also a transport mechanism to release toxins from the body, heat speeds up and enhances this process. The skin is the largest organ of detoxification, and allowing it to sweat out its impurities is a great benefit to health.

6) Lactic acid dispersed

A useful benefit of saunas and steam rooms in exercise facilities is that they help the body to disperse lactic acid from the muscles. During heavy exercise the muscles can run out of glucose – their main fuel sources – and instead go into anaerobic respiration to generate energy. This type of energy creates lactic acid as a byproduct which can build up in the body and cause sore muscles the day after exercising. A heat treatment following exercise can help lessen or remove this effect.

7) Heart rate

Heat treatments have been long proven to give clients the equivalent of a mild cardiovascular workout, and are excellent for everyday fitness. As the body dilates capillaries and drives blood to the surface of the skin the heart beats faster in order to pump blood more effectively to the extremities. During this process the faster heartbeat strengthens the heart in a muscular sense in the same way as swimming or brisk walking might.

8) Pores open

The first flush of a heat treatment opens up the pores of the body to eliminate toxins. This exposes the skin to a deeper level of cleansing than is usually achieved in a shower. Ongoing conditions such as acne can also benefit from the pore-opening properties of heat treatments.

Similarly the cleansed pores and skin allow proceeding treatments such as wraps and masks to be more effective and penetrate the skin more readily.

9) Skin is softened

Skin becomes softer, and this can allow better and easier treatment which focuses on areas of the body where hard skin has formed. In particular pedicures will benefit from heat treatment, allowing the softened skin on the heels and balls of the feet to be more readily sloughed away and moisturised.

10) Sebaceous gland activity is increased

Sebaceous glands secrete a natural oily waxy substance – sebum, designed to moisturise and protect the skin. It is thought by many to be one of the skin's best moisturisers as it is naturally occurring. Additionally, whilst sufferers of excess sebum production may fear this effect, the result is actually balancing for the skin.

11) Metabolic rate increases

Heat increases the metabolic rate as the body cools itself, increasing the heart rate and generation of energy. This has a positive effect for weight-loss purposes as stored fuels such as fat are more readily burned for energy. The effect of speeding the metabolism can last for several hours following treatment.

12) Blood pressure falls

As moisture and toxins evaporate from the body, blood pressure falls. The result is less pressure on the cardiovascular system with reduced potential damage to arteries and capillaries.

13) Lymphatic drainage is increased

As the heart rate increases and the circulation around the body increases, lymphatic drainage is enhanced. The lymphatic system works in parallel with the circulatory system and is driven by muscular contractions and the opening and closing of valves. As one function of the lymph is to drain away waste materials this has a beneficial effect on the removal of toxins from the body, although adequate hydration is essential.

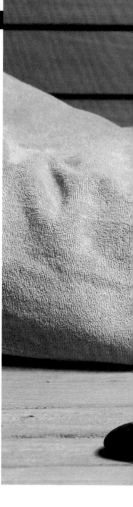

Endpoints
By the end of this topic, you should understand:

- the advantages and benefits of heat therapy
- potential applications of these advantages to treatment
- possibilities of combining heat treatments with other treatments for optimal effect.

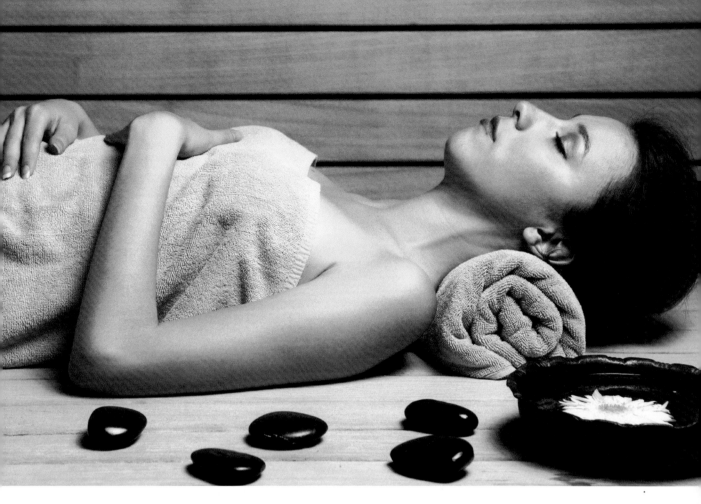

TOPIC 2: HEAT AND HYDRATION

The effect of heat in and on the body is greatly dependent on issues of hydration. This can refer to both the moisture content of the heat used as well as the hydration levels of the individual receiving treatment.

TYPES OF HEAT

Generally there are two types of heat found in a treatment setting – moist heat or dry heat. Both work on the principles of cleansing by perspiration.

Moist heat

This is the kind of heat found in steam rooms, where moist water is heated to evaporate into the air. Those who find the dry heat environment of a sauna too uncomfortable may prefer the more gentle feel of moist heat.

• KEY POINT

The levels of humidity, or moisture content of the air will greatly affect how a particular temperature feels to the body.

Main factors of moist heat:

- Gentle feeling of heat on the skin.
- Temperature 180F to 235F.
- Can be pleasantly fragranced.
- Used in steam rooms in 'hammam' style Turkish baths.
- Often large facilities with plenty of space.
- Also used in small fibreglass units for one person only.

Dry heat

The dry heat of sauna's may feel hotter to clients, but it is in fact generally a cooler heat than that found in steam rooms.

Main factors of dry heat:

- Effective at drawing sweat from the body and creating rapid heat sensation.
- Temperature 110F to 130F.
- Used in wooden saunas of Nordic style.
- Can fit in very small spaces, and can comprise a single bench.

• DID YOU KNOW?

Saunas have long hailed from very cold countries such as Sweden and Finland as being excellent for the health. In ancient times some women even chose to give birth in the sauna!

CLIENT HYDRATION LEVELS

The effect of heat treatments on the body is very beneficial. But managing a client's hydration levels is essential to getting the most from a heat treatment.

In hot conditions the body will sweat more freely, driving out toxins, but water will also be lost from the skin in this process. Sauna conditions can cause the body to lose between half a litre (one pints) and a litre (two pints) of water quite rapidly. However, this is also replaced very quickly when the client rehydrates by drinking water.

Optimal hydration levels

A correctly hydrated body should be between 60-70% water. This figure can be calculated using electronic scales, as discussed in Chapter 2: Body analysis.

Hydration levels for the average person are suboptimal at around 50%, which means that even before entering a heat treatment facility clients should be encouraged to drink water or a fruit or herbal tea.

Adipose influence on dehydration

Excess fat (or adipose tissue) means the body has less facility to store water, as fat cells hold only

• KEY POINT

Clients undergoing heat treatment should always have access to drinking water facilities.

• KEY POINT

A correctly hydrated kidney can effectively excrete its toxic load, efficiently flushing out the body and enhancing the effects of heat treatment.

15% water in contrast to the 75% held by muscle cells.

This means that clients carrying excess fat will be less able to stay well hydrated, even if they consume large amounts of water. For this reason clients in this category should be more closely monitored in heated conditions for symptoms of heat exhaustion or illness, as described in Chapter 4: Tanning. Similarly, highly muscular clients have a higher tolerance in heated conditions.

BENEFITS OF OPTIMAL HYDRATION WITH HEAT TREATMENT

The benefits of heat treatment are greatly enhanced by optimal hydration, and some benefits of heat can even be reversed by poor hydration.

1) Kidneys

The kidneys judge when the body is dehydrated via pressure and salt sensitive cells. In this circumstance they secrete hormones which reabsorb more salt from the body into the blood stream and this has the effect of drawing more water into the blood.

The net result is that less water is lost from the kidneys into the urine. However, the kidneys also excrete water-soluble toxins, and are reliant on adequate hydration to perform this task optimally. In circumstances where the body is dehydrated less toxins are able to be excreted by the kidney. This negative consequence is further exacerbated in heated conditions where more toxins are being urged through the system by a faster metabolism and heartbeat.

2) Lymphatic system

The lymphatic system drains excess fluids from the tissues of the body, and carries toxic waste to be excreted. This process is enhanced by optimal hydration which helps maintain balance within the lymphatic system.

3) Blood pressure

Dehydration lowers blood pressure by removing liquid from the blood. The body is able to counter this effect with proper hydration, and benefits of low blood pressure will be conferred. If hydration is very poor, the resulting dehydration can cause dizziness or even fainting.

4) Sweating

Heat treatments increase perspiration thereby increasing the excretion of toxins via the skin. Correct levels of hydration help and support this process, providing plenty of fluid with which the water-soluble toxins can be flushed out of the skin.

4) Excess hydration

Whilst water is lost during heat treatment, salt and other electrolytes are also expelled from the skin. For this reason it is very important not to over-hydrate. Excess water consumption combined with loss of electrolytes can critically affect the body's natural electrical currents which function in brain activity and muscle contractions. No more than three large glasses of filtered water should be drunk proceeding treatment.

• DID YOU KNOW?

Ideal blood pressure is at or below 120 over 80 (120/80).

Endpoints

By the end of this topic, you should understand:

- the difference between wet and dry heat
- common places wet and dry heat are used, and usual characteristics of the different heat
- importance of keeping clients hydrated during treatment
- effects of hydration on the body's capacity to detoxify and deal with heat.

TOPIC 3: HEAT TREATMENT FACILITIES

Heat treatments can take various different forms, from heated rooms to more direct application. As a spa therapist you may have access to several different means of administering heat treatments for your clients.

SAUNA

Saunas are of Nordic or Finnish origin, and are comprised of an insulated room made of pine wood which is heated using internal coals. The wooden interior is lined on the outside with a very effective insulating material, and then a further 'skin' of pine wood. Inside stones or smokeless coals are heated to a very high temperature by an electric heater, providing a dry heat. A wooden bucket and wooden ladle are provided in order to douse the stones with water. This releases a surge of heat as the moist air rises and is absorbed by the wood walls.

Pine is used to both absorb moisture and provide a pleasant scent which many believe is good for the lungs. The wood interior also helps to radiate the heat back out into the cabin. For this reason saunas are very versatile, and can be built to stand alone in a variety of spaces.

• KEY POINT

Very small saunas can be built the size of a large shower cubicle, making them a practical option even for facilities with limited space.

Practicalities

The thermostat for temperature adjustment is usually situated outside of the cabin to prevent inappropriate adjustment by the client.

Different levels of seating in the sauna allow different temperatures to be enjoyed. Higher levels confer stronger heat.

No metal of any kind should ever be taken inside the sauna, as it will heat to a temperature which could cause burns.

Infrared saunas

These are saunas which are heated by infra-red light rather than an electric heater. They carry almost all the same structural properties of a regular sauna, being made of an insulated box of pine wood, with tiered seating to allow clients access to varying heat.

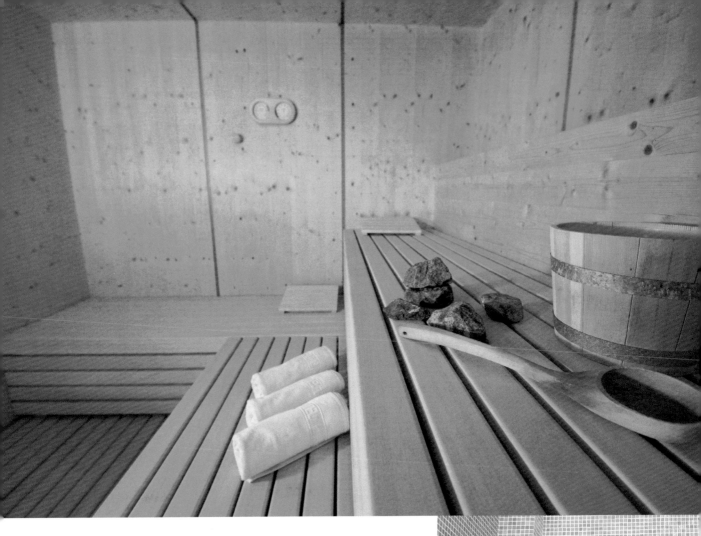

Rather than heat which is absorbed indirectly through warm air, however, infrared energy is absorbed directly into the body from lights situated throughout the sauna. Infrared is a type of light energy which is part of the electromagnetic spectrum (see Chapter 4: Tanning for more on this), and is thought by some to offer more effective muscle soothing for clients with conditions such as arthritis.

Infrared saunas remove more body impurities at lower temperatures than traditional heat treatments. Healthy infrared light gently warms the body without over-heating the air around, meaning clients enjoy the health benefits associated with a sauna session in a drier, cooler atmosphere than traditional saunas.

STEAM BATH/ROOMS

In its traditional form, steam baths comprise an entire facility in their own right, and are still found in this form in countries such as Turkey and Morocco. These very large baths can be comprised of a number of rooms of varying temperatures. The

● DID YOU KNOW?

Saunas always come equipped with an internal thermometer which will clearly show if the heat inside is too hot or too cool. If you find a facility with no thermometer you should immediately alert a person in charge.

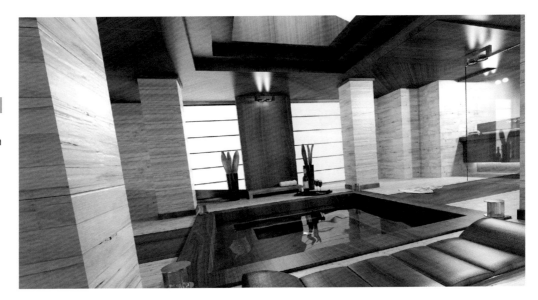

DID YOU KNOW?

The steam bath is also known as a hammam in Morroco, and a banya in Russia.

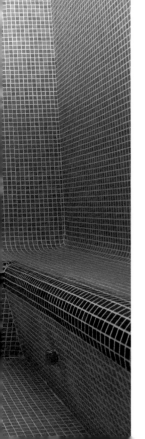

premise of the more basic of these baths is as a community washing facility, and separate rooms for men and women to soap and clean themselves among friends. More modern facilities also incorporate treatments and massage.

In western spas, steam baths are more likely to take the form of a standalone room.

Within the facility scented steam can be provided, and the steam room is often a precursor to the stronger heat of the sauna.

Steam cabinets

These are steam baths engineered for a single person, and take the form of a large cabinet, usually made from fibre glass. They can also be referred to as steam baths. The client enters the cabinet which is closed around their body with a seat inside, and a space for their head at the top. Towels are placed to shield where the client's neck could make contact with the cabinet. Inside a zippered plastic covering is placed around the client to facilitate sweating, whilst at the base a heated container of water causes steam to rise upwards.

Clients must be supervised whilst in steam cabinets in case the heat overwhelms them.

Cabinets can be manufactured from fibreglass or metal. Metal cabinets are hard-wearing and cost-effective, but harder to clean, require more protective towels, and are less attractive looking.

Clients should be shown how they may leave the steam cabinet unaided. The door normally opens outwards so they can walk out easily

The internal temperature should be 45-50C.

PLUNGE POOLS

Plunge pools are popular teamed with saunas rather than steam baths, as the intense heat of the former lends itself better to rapid cooling. Some facilities have very cold plunge pools, and in Nordic regions some saunas are even matched with a frozen lake with a cut out section for freezing plunges. In modern facilities, however, cool rather than cold is usually preferable. Some modern spa facilities use the milder temperature of a swimming pool for this purpose.

Extreme cold and extreme heat can have some benefits to the circulation, but these are best applied as a managed treatment under the guidance of a therapist.

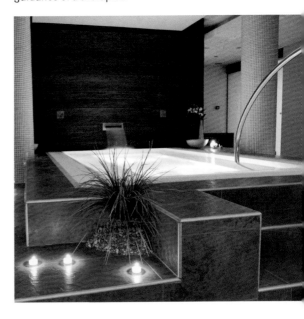

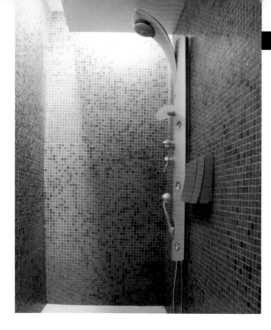

• KEY POINT

Never assume that your client will know what to expect. Clear guidance throughout their spa experience is essential.

SHOWERS

A facility which provides sauna or steam room treatment should have sufficient showers and clients should be directed to use these before heat treatments. This will help keep equipment clean, and will enable a better result in terms of skin health.

Special showers, however, are sometimes provided for the purpose of dousing with cold water. These are usually located immediately outside the sauna or steam room. Variations on these can include buckets of cold water, which can then be emptied over the head for maximum impact. Some saunas even provide ice for clients to rub over their bodies following a treatment.

For the purposes of relaxation and preparation for additional treatments, however, tepid showers are the best choice for clients between sauna exposures.

ETIQUETTE

Clients are often unsure as to the etiquette for saunas and steam rooms, as the practice varies internationally, and even from spa to spa.

In the UK and the US standard practice is to enter the sauna in full swimwear, or covered with a towel. In Eastern Europe and Scandinavia, however, any clothing in a sauna is considered inappropriate.

Client comfort is of paramount importance. They should be given clear directions as to what to expect during a spa visit. In the case of steam cabinets a therapist will be on hand to guide the client through the procedure, but with saunas and steam rooms which clients access themselves, clear instructions are normally located within the treatment area.

HYGIENE

Due to the perspiration which takes place in heated facilities, particular care should be taken to regularly clean, sanitise/sterilise and maintain equipment. Clean towels and robes should be provided for each client. Heated conditions are perfect breeding grounds for bacteria, and facilities should be rigorously monitored for this reason.

CHECKLIST
- Treatment areas and equipment should be cleaned with sanitising/sterilising solution daily.
- Ensure benches are covered with clean paper towels for each client.
- Ensure the client showers before entering the treatment area and that swimwear or similar is worn.
- Ensure that there are clean towels and robes available for each client.

Endpoints

By the end of this topic, you should understand:
- **the different types of heated equipment used such as saunas and steam baths**
- **subsets of these types of equipment**
- **additional equipment found alongside heated treatment facilities, such as rapid-cooling devices**
- **etiquette for saunas and steam baths**
- **hygiene requirements for heat treatment equipment.**

TOPIC 4:
CONTRAINDICATIONS

Heat treatments should be used with caution and in particular where open flames or hot coals are involved. You should follow general health and safety guidelines as laid out in Chapter 1, but in addition you should be aware of particular contraindications which relate to heat treatments.

Heated conditions can be dangerous, and therapists should be aware of the symptoms of heat exhaustion and similar heat-related illness

As a professional therapist you must always make sure that a consultation is carried out prior to treatment and that any contraindications are documented. Contraindications can be classified into those that require medical, GP or specialist permission and those that restrict or prohibit treatment.

In circumstances where written medical permission cannot be obtained the client must sign an informed consent stating that the treatment and its effects has been fully explained to them and confirm that they are willing to proceed without permission from their GP or specialist.

Conditions which may be treated with medical consent include:
- Pregnancy
- Cardio vascular conditions (thrombosis, phlebitis, hypertension, hypotension, heart conditions)
- Haemophilia (a genetic condition which interferes with blood clotting)
- Medical oedema (water retention)
- Osteoporosis (bone thinning)
- Arthritis (or similar joint pain)
- Nervous/psychotic conditions
- Epilepsy
- Recent operations
- Diabetes
- Asthma
- Any dysfunction of the nervous system (e.g. muscular sclerosis, Parkinson's disease, motor neurone disease)
- Bells palsy
- Trapped/pinched nerve (e.g. sciatica)
- Inflamed nerve
- Cancer
- Postural deformities
- Spastic conditions
- Kidney infections
- Whiplash
- Slipped disc
- Undiagnosed pain
- When taking prescribed medication
- Acute rheumatism
- Any condition already being treated by a GP or another complementary practitioner.

Contraindications which may restrict treatment
Other conditions restrict or prohibit treatment entirely. The following conditions should never be exposed to heat treatment.
- Fever
- Contagious or infectious diseases
- Under the influence of recreational drugs or alcohol
- Diarrhoea and vomiting
- Skin diseases
- Localised swelling
- Recent fractures (minimum three months)
- Cervical spondylitis
- Undiagnosed lumps and bumps
- Inflammation
- Varicose veins
- Cuts
- Bruises
- Abrasions
- Scar tissues (two years for major operation and

six months for a small scar)
- Sunburn
- Hormonal implants
- First few days of menstruation depending how the client feels
- Haematoma
- Hernia
- Recent fractures (minimum three months)
- Cervical spondylitis
- Gastric ulcers
- After a heavy meal
- Conditions affecting the neck.

If the client has any other condition which you are unsure about, always insist they consult with their doctor or sign an informed consent form before performing heat treatment.

HEALTH AND SAFETY CHECKLIST
- Ensure that the treatment is explained to the client before commencement.
- Ensure the correct temperature is adhered to.
- Check temperature gauge.
- Ensure the client stays in the sauna/steam room for maximum ten mins .
- After ten mins they should take a warm shower or plunge in a warm pool (not freezing).
- They may repeat the process a number of times.
- Ensure the client drinks plenty of water.
- Ensure that the client rests in the rest area and allows the body temperature to return to normal before leaving the spa.

TOPIC 5: AFTERCARE

Heat treatments often form a valuable precursor to other relaxing treatments, but they can also be used as a treatment in their own right. Clients may enjoy a day at a spa, for example, simply using heat treatment equipment without any additional treatments.

Depending on whether a treatment is administered after heat therapy, aftercare will vary slightly, but the basic proponents remain the same.

Shower
Skin exposed to heat treatment will be doused in a mix of water, salt and other toxins, and these should be removed from the body.

Hydrate
Hydration before and after heat treatment is important, but spa therapists will usually be in a better position to offer water or herbal teas proceeding a treatment. Clients should sip rather than gulp up to three glasses of room temperature water.

Moisturise
Skin exposed to heat will be bathed in sweat which can have levels of acidity which strips the skin of moisture. Additionally, the removal of the natural oils combined with the deep cleansing effect of the heat on the pores can leave skin dry.

It may be that the client has enjoyed heat treatment as a precursor to another therapy such as a body mask, wrap or massage, in which case the resulting oils and lotions will serve to moisturise the skin. But if the client is leaving immediately after a treatment they should be advised to moisturise as soon as possible.

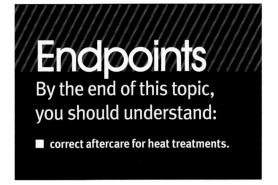

Endpoints
By the end of this topic, you should understand:

- **correct aftercare for heat treatments.**

06

Spas

Professional spas offer total relaxation and are the ultimate in therapeutic escape. The services on offer range from on-off treatments to full managed retreats, but always in a specialist environment carefully designed to delight and soothe the senses.

Understanding the spa setting means knowing about the origins of the concept, and the aspects which are generally understood to comprise a spa. You must recognise the high professional standards expected of these luxury facilities, and have specialist knowledge of working in a water-based environment.

In this chapter we'll be looking at the following key topics to understand more about the spa concept and professional care of spa areas.

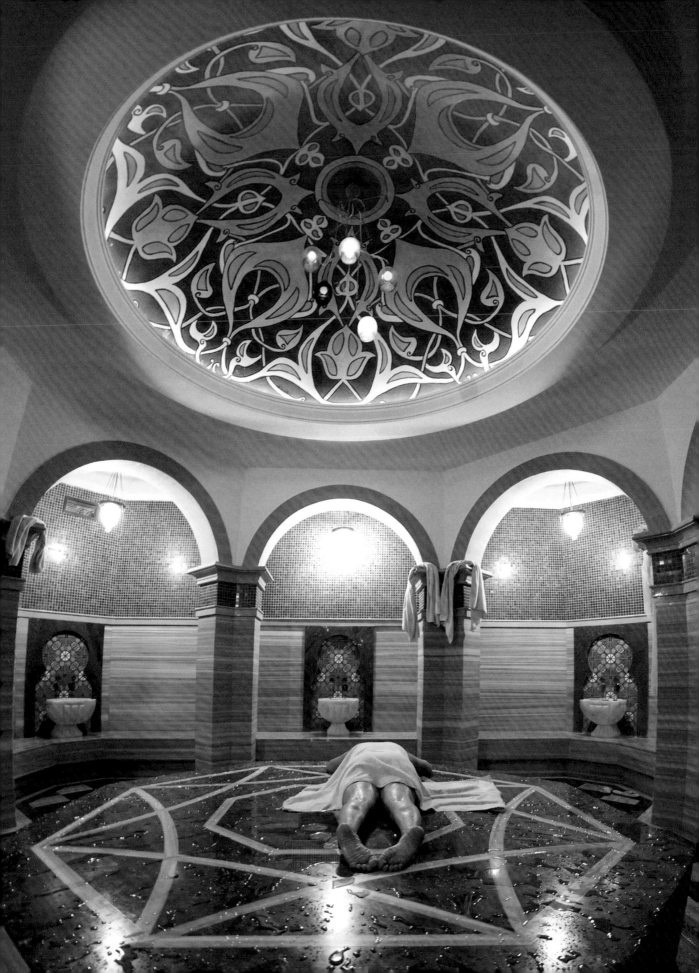

TOPIC 1:
THE SPA CONCEPT

Whilst many people feel they have an understanding of what a spa is, the actual concept is quite rigidly defined. During this topic we'll learn about the origins of the modern day spa, as well the criteria by which they are generally understood.

The history of the spa

Spa services have come a long way since their origins many hundreds of years ago. The first spas were often located at the site of naturally occurring springs or lakes which were thought to offer healing waters, and people travelled hundreds of miles to enjoy rejuvenation or alleviate health conditions. Historically, famous spas were places like Lourdes in France, where the water was believed to be imbued with holy qualities which could cure illness. In England, Bath was a popular destination for aristocrats to 'take the waters' in the eighteenth century.

• KEY POINT

The term spa is often used to denote any area which offers therapeutic services. As we will come to explore, however, a professional spa is a much more comprehensive definition.

In the twentieth century, spas began to take on a new meaning. They became more comprehensive places for people to relax and take treatments designed for health. With their history as places of healing, these early spas still had a definite medical slant and surroundings were clinical rather than calming.

As time has progressed and celebrity culture has taken hold, aristocrats have been replaced with wealthy stars, who are interested in treatments for beauty as well as health. The environments have evolved to become places where those with pressured lives can wind down, and this theme has

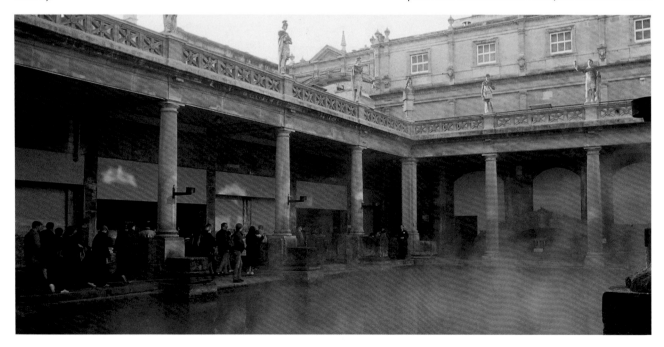

continued towards the modern day as spas have become available to more ordinary people as well as the rich and famous.

The five senses

The millennial spa is a haven for the senses and must appeal to all elements of touch, taste, sight, sound and smell to be truly considered a spa.

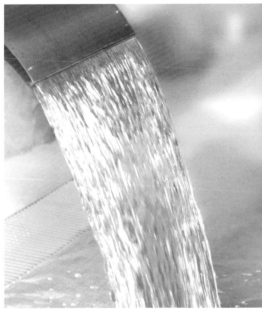

1) Sight

Soft colours, mood lighting and ambiance are all factors when designing a spa. The best in the world put an enormous amount of effort into designing imaginative spaces of soothing light and interiors designed to complement the flow of water. Natural elements such as wood and stone are often put to great effect to lift the client from the pressures of their modern day life and create a dreamlike world of relaxation.

As a therapist your spa will have been designed for your professional use, but within this space it is your job to continue to maintain the spa environment ensures a luxury experience for your client. A good spa will be impeccably maintained with flawless hygiene and perfect order. This is a space in which people will be able to relax and release their daily cares, and your responsibility is to keep this environment as it has been designed.

• DID YOU KNOW?

Technically a spa should have access to its own pure running water source to meet the terminology. But modern day facilities allow for some leeway.

2) Sound

Many spas rely on the sound of running water to add a background ambiance to their more public spaces. In private therapy rooms it is usual practice to provide gentle instrumental music, or to use soundtracks of natural settings such as forests or ocean waves.

Volume is also important, as even the most soothing of music can become intrusive if played too loud.

For the same reason noise levels in the spa in general should be kept to a minimum. Speak softly and monitor situations in which noise could disturb your clients. During the planning period it would also be wise to ensure that the general passageways and maintenance areas (laundry, dispensaries) are kept away from the treatments areas as it can be disturbing for clients who are trying to optimise the time to relax.

3) Smell

All spas should smell attractive, and often this is part of the subconscious journey into relaxation. A client may not actively realise that they have

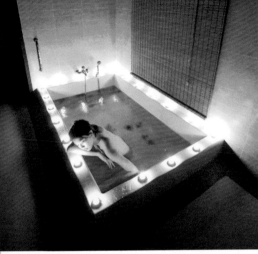

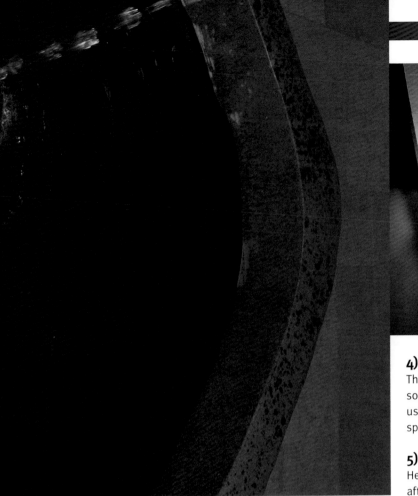

4) Touch

This usually forms part of the spa treatment via the soothing hands of the therapist. In addition care is usually taken to ensure the physical environs of the spa are pleasingly comfortable to relax in.

5) Taste

Herbal and fruit teas are often served before and after therapies and are an ideal method with which to help hydrate the client following a treatment. If possible there should always be facilities to offer clients a drink of this sort as they are waiting for treatments, and whilst they are relaxing afterwards.

A word about the five senses

Most spas strive to achieve the delight of all five senses, but just as important as meeting every single criteria is the creation of a balanced, relaxing and sensual environment.

walked into a pleasantly fragranced environment, but proper use of aromatherapy will assure them they are entering a different world. In the public areas spas tend to use perfumes which are delicate yet uplifting such as orange blossom or bergamot. In the treatment rooms a more restful fragrance is used.

Aromatherapy candles or oil burners can be used for this purpose, although utmost care must be taken with health and safety regarding open flames. More practical for the busy spa are electronic diffusers which can waft scent using a fan and filters, or oil diffusing wooden sticks which have the added advantage of being silent.

Uplifting fragrances

Citrus scents such as orange, lemon, bergamot or a blend of these is perfect for welcoming clients into the spa area.

Relaxing fragrances

Soothing scents such as lavender, ylang ylang and rose are good choices for treatment rooms.

Endpoints
By the end of this topic, you should understand:

■ the history of the spa
■ what a modern day spa delivers
■ how to address meeting the 'five senses' experience of sight, sound, taste, touch and smell.

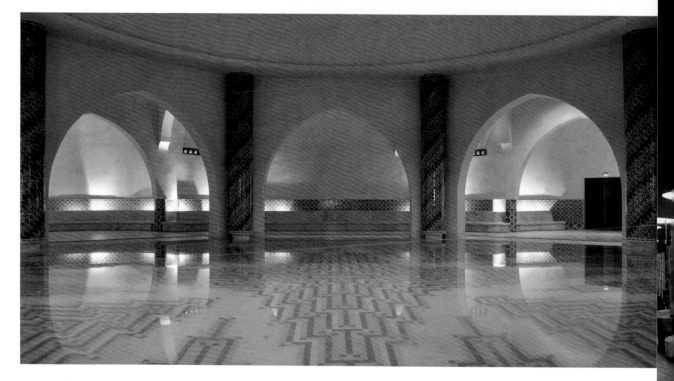

TOPIC 2:
TYPES OF SPA

There are many different types of spa, and amongst these types treatments will vary, although there is often a degree of overlap. From very large resort spas to smaller outlets there is room for variation in size, but as we will come to discover, certain standards must be reached to truly earn the title.

The destination spa –

- Clients book in for time periods spanning from a few days, weeks or even months.
- Spa offers accommodation.
- The environment is designed to facilliate longer treatment programmes.

This is the traditional 'rich and famous' retreat, used to revitalise, detoxify and undertake weight management programmes.

Within this category there are varying methods, with some offering regimented 'juice diets' or similarly restrictive programmes, whilst others simply provide an environment where low calorie meals are teamed with exercise sessions and treatments.

• KEY POINT

The term 'spa' can relate to many different types of establishment, from a day spa offering treatments to a destination spa where clients could stay for many days, weeks or months.

Often a client can pick or choose the exact elements of their stay, but all will be available for the designated stay with a specific goal, whether to lose a certain amount of weight, or to optimise health.

The latest version of this kind of spa is the 'bootcamp' whereby clients engage in rigorous daily exercise teamed with low calorie meals. For the most part, however, therapists will be working in destination spas of a more gentle kind with treatments to complement healthy activities.

These spas are not open to the general public and must be booked in advance for a designated amount of time.

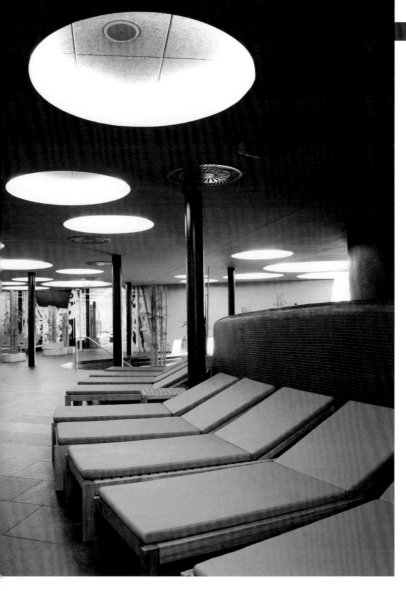

The day spa

■ Likely to be attached to a gym or health centre and what used to be known as Beauty salons.

■ Offers treatments which can be combined with use of other facilities.

■ Ideal for short treatments.

These spas have become increasingly popular, and unfortunately are the source of much confusion as to how the term 'spa' should be used. 'Day spa' is wrongly applied to many facilities which cannot claim to offer the full sensual experience of a destination spa, such as gyms or beauty salons which merely include extra treatments such as massage, wraps and masks.

Generally to be classed as a day spa a venue must offer an extensive complement of full body treatments, facials and aromatherapy with professional spa products. The environment must meet the expected criteria of appealing to the five senses and include showering and changing facilities for both sexes and bathrobes.

Medical spas

■ Usually offer accommodation for clients.

■ Often offer unique treatments for specific medical conditions as well as general health.

■ Popular with older clients.

In general medical spas are more popular on the Continent and particularly towards Eastern Europe where medical massages combine with water treatments. They can also be destinations which are combined with aesthetic surgical procedures in order to afford recovery time in relaxed and private environments particularly popular in the USA, South Africa and Australia.

The resort spa

■ Commonly found as part of luxury hotel accommodation.

■ Large variation in size and facilities.

■ Designed to provide further relaxation resources for those holidaying.

This spa may be attached to a hotel or resort. Due to the space available these spas come in different shapes and sizes, with some able to devote large spaces and outdoor areas to their spas whilst others are limited to a few treatment rooms by the pool area.

These smaller spas are known as 'amenity spas' which extend from an existing pool area or work-out space with a la carte services.

Larger resort spas offer treatment packages alongside a dedicated spa space with changing rooms.

● DID YOU KNOW?

Whilst the concept of spas is now international, there are still some marked variations in trends across the world. Whilst countries such as the UK and the US are likely to have similar spas, areas such as Switzerland have developed their own form of treatments which have different criteria. In general medical spas are more likely to be found in Eastern Europe and Switzerland. However the modern trends are medical spas more likely to be found in the USA, South Africa and Australia where clients convalesce after cosmetic surgery whilst receiving spa and skin rejuvenating treatments'.

CHECKLIST – WHAT IS A SPA

To meet the accepted criteria to be designated a spa the following standards must be met:

- ☐ Stimulation of the 'five senses' (touch, taste, sound, smell and sight) must comprise part of the experience.
- ☐ A clean and nurturing environment.
- ☐ Correct laundered robes and towels for all sizes.
- ☐ Showering and changing facilities for both sexes.
- ☐ Professional products either in the spa's name or another quality brand which staff are trained to use.
- ☐ Massages, body treatments (such as wraps and masks), facials and aromatherapy expertise must be available.
- ☐ Hydrotherapy treatment such as whirlpools, hot tubs and floatation.
- ☐ Lockers or facilities for clients to store their valuables.

Endpoints

By the end of this topic, you should understand:

- ■ the concept of different types of spas available to clients
- ■ an overview of what kinds of spa might be suitable for which treatments
- ■ the basic criteria of what defines a spa.

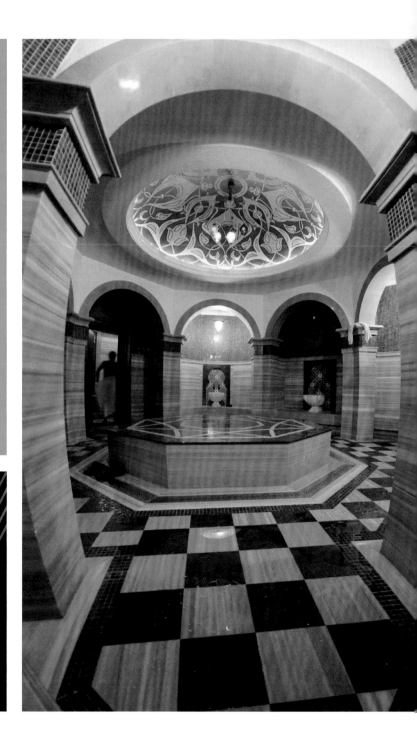

TOPIC 3: AREAS WITHIN THE SPA

Modern day spas can be very large, containing numerous areas for treatment, from wet rooms to relaxing pool and sauna areas. Each element comes with its own criteria and code of conduct for professional maintenance.

The spa reception area

This is the client's first experience of the spa, and their personal greeting is just as important as the physical environment they are entering. The reception area should be calming and inviting, and those welcoming clients should be well presented and smiling.

Any materials which the clients use to sign in should be readily available as well as neat and clean. Plentiful lists of treatments available should be on hand for clients to browse as well as printed materials for them to take away. The reception area should be manned at all times.

The wet area

Spas are usually comprise of an extensive 'wet' area which contain potential hazards such as slippery tiled surfaces. These should be free from excessive water to avoid slippages and cleansed regularly. They often house the steam, sauna and whirlpool/hot tub and are sometimes linked to either a swimming pool or large hydrotherapy pool area.

The wet room is an area in which hydrotherapy treatments can be administered. It is a tiled room with a suitably waterproof treatment bed, taps, showers and hoses as needed and correct drainage facilities to allow removal of water.

Spa pool/hot tub

A Jacuzzi is the original (branded) name for a spa pool and is also known as a hot tub. It is kept at a warm 38-41C, around the temperature of a cooler bath. Air is pumped through into the water by jets creating massage conditions underneath the water.

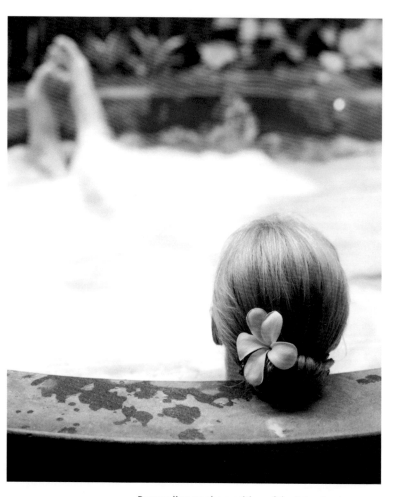

Depending on the position of the jets clients can align themselves for stronger or milder massage by the water.

A sauna is a heated wooden unit in which clients can attain heightened body temperature to

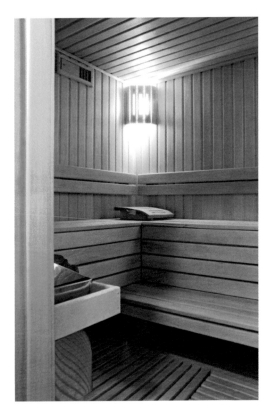

In the UK and the US standard practice is to enter the sauna in full swimwear, or covered with a towel. In Eastern Europe and Scandinavia, however, any clothing in a sauna is inappropriate, and thought to interfere with breathing. For this reason it is sensible to ensure signs are posted indicating which conditions are expected in the sauna.

harsh on their lungs a steam room can offer a gentle alternative. Alternatively the steam room and sauna can be used in combination one after the other (repeating as many times as the client wishes) in addition to or as part of a bespoke treatment plan.

A larger style steam room is also known as a hammam or a Turkish bath. Some spas have these but they are still more commonly found in the Middle East as a stand-alone facility with treatment rooms attached.

Changing rooms

These are subject to the usual health and safety cautions of any area exposed to water regularly. Lockers and showers are usually provided within the changing rooms.

Laundry facilities

Every spa should have a full complement of clean and freshly laundered towels and robes available for clients of every size.

Relaxation area/room

Not all spas have a dedicated room for relaxation, but this room, when provided should be kept as an oasis of calm. Soothing music, comfortable furnishings, and low lighting are vital aspects. If you work in a spa it can be easy to overlook the relaxation area. If you can, make it a regularly practice to sit as if you were a client in the room to notice any aspects which may have been overlooked.

induce healthy sweating. If saunas are for general use (rather than specific treatments) care must be undertaken to ensure clients are made aware of the cultural expectations of dress within this environment. Saunas are covered in more detail in Chapter 5.

There are differing ways of providing heat in a sauna:

- Swedish style sauna – this is the kind commonly found in spas. Heat is provided from coals which can be splashed with water to provide extra heat.
- Infra-red sauna – these saunas need extra time to be heated in advance of use and heat the environment using infra red beams.
- Smoke-sauna – these saunas are heated using wood-smoke for several hours and then the smoke is vented through the ceiling. They are popular in cold climates.

Steam rooms offer a more humid version of the sauna, often with a more gentle heat. For some clients who feel the dry air of the sauna is

Endpoints

By the end of this topic, you should understand:

- modern day spas can consist of many different areas
- which areas are appropriate for which task or treatment
- basic expectations of professional practice in different areas of the spa.

TOPIC 4: THE SPA ENVIRONMENT

Due to its nature as a wet environment the spa has a number of elements which should be considered for client comfort which makes the distinction between a spa and a typical treatment room.

The elements of the five senses should be considered when administering any treatment, but in regards to the spa environment there are additional important factors which should be understood.

Temperature –

It is impossible for a client to relax in conditions which are too cold. Not only will they feel less inclined to remove clothing for a treatment but their muscles will be rigid and body language closed. For this reason spas are usually heated slightly hotter than usual workplaces to aid relaxation. A simple wall-mounted thermometer can be used to judge temperature.

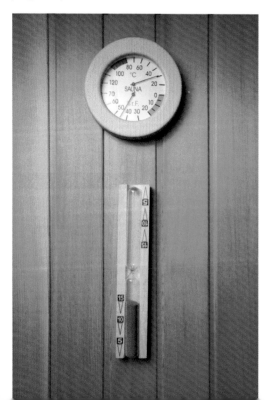

• DID YOU KNOW?

According to The UK Workplace Regulations 1992 no professional environment should fall below 19C. For most spas, however this is several degrees too cool, and a more usual temperature would be between 25-28C. This applies to all areas of the spa, including changing rooms and therapy rooms.

Humidity

By their nature, spas are humid environments and this actually confers health benefits in terms of respiration and skin. For very humid environments, however humidifiers can be purchased and the humidity in general should be monitored for comfort. Remember that if you are working in a spa daily you will adjust to the various conditions, so take any feedback from clients very seriously. Electronic meters can be used to measure humidity which are inexpensive and readily available.

- Humidity refers to the amount of water vapour in the air.
- Warm air can hold more water, so because they use warm water spas usually have high humidity.
- Humidity is measured as a percentage, and anything above 65% can be considered humid.

Ventilation

Ventilation must be adequate and designed for optimal relaxation and comfort. In general a breeze is not appropriate which can make it easy to overlook ventilation. This makes it even more important to ensure ventilation equipment is operating as it should and is regularly serviced. Malfunctioning air-conditioning equipment can impart an unpleasant damp odour and poorly ventilated rooms can create hygiene issues.

Waste disposal
Equipment

As with any therapeutic environment you will most likely be disposing of large quantities of waste products which have been used during treatments.

In a spa environment, however, this waste will take the form of larger items for disposal and a greater quantity of wet products. This might include plastic wraps which have been used to apply a full-body mud mask, or the cleaning of hot towels which have been used to remove a product from a client's body.

Ensure you have adequate facilities to dispose of or cleanse items before carrying out a treatment, and remember that a client should never see items for waste disposal.

Water

Dirty water will also comprise an important area of waste to be considered and adequate facilities should be provided for its correct disposal. Any water which has been in contact with human bodies can be considered contaminated, and treatment water should never be reused.

Endpoints
By the end of this topic, you should understand:

- the key environmental 'comfort factors' such as heat and humidity in a spa
- equipment used to help monitor and moderate conditions within the spa.
- the importance of proper waste and water disposal.

TOPIC 5: WATER HEALTH AND SAFETY

Water is put to great use in spas for the purposes of relaxation and administering treatments. This does, however, mean that much care needs to be taken to ensure that issues of hygiene and safety are properly addressed. In keeping water clean, strong chemicals are used which themselves can be hazardous and must be treated with the utmost respect.

Water levels

When using equipment such as hot tubs and pools the water levels should be carefully monitored. Hot tubs in particular will have a waterline below which the contents should not fall, and to allow the equipment to sink below this could cause very expensive damage.

The waterline around the rim of the pool or tub will also build up dirt which must be cleansed regularly using specialist cleaning fluids. This is most likely to be left to specialist cleaning staff, but you should be aware of possible issues.

Water hygiene

Keeping the water clean is the most important part of maintaining a spa environment. Warm water such as that found in hot tubs and spa pools makes the perfect breeding grounds for bacteria, particularly when mixed with the debris of skin cells, oils, dirt and other contaminants from usage by bathers.

• KEY POINT

Water can be very dangerous if not properly supervised, and care should always be taken in environments where it is used for part of treatments, or for bathing and relaxing.

Three steps to perfect spa water –
These can be remembered as ABC reversed –
so CBA are your three steps.

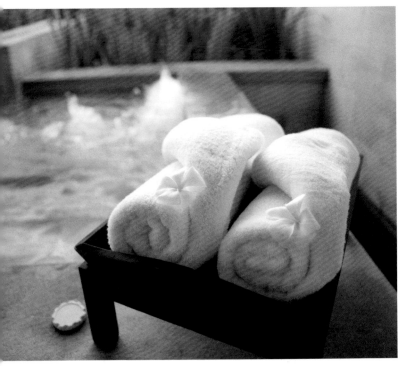

Clean
Clean spa water by using a professional sanitising agent such as chlorine or bromine. Generally bromine is more appropriate for a spa or small pool such as a hot tub, since it has a less intrusive odour than chlorine and is longer lasting as a disinfectant. As it is more expensive as a hygiene agent than chlorine it is not generally used for larger pool areas.

Break down debris
This is sometimes known as 'shock treatment' and is usually performed around once a week. Once the chlorine or bromine has neutralised bacteria the resulting residue needs to be broken down which will then allow the pool filtration system to remove it.

Alkaline balance
Spa water must be at the right pH level. This means it is not too acidic or not too alkaline, but perfectly balanced for skin comfort.

• KEY POINT
PH level is the name of the scale on which acid or alkaline is rated. The scale ranges from one to fourteen.

The pH scale –
A liquid is defined as acid or alkaline by the number of free hydrogen ions found in a concentration of fluid.

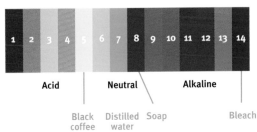

Acid
Lots of hydrogen ions make a low pH or acidic substance.
■ An acid substance scores between one and six.
■ A strongly acidic substance is stomach acid with a pH of one.
■ Less acidic is black coffee, with a pH of five.
■ Acid is corrosive, and in a spa environment acidic water can corrode and damage expensive equipment such as pipes and filters, and can irritate skin.

Neutral
■ A balanced number of hydrogen ions make a neutral pH.
■ A neutral substance is defined as scoring seven on the pH scale.
■ Distilled water is defined as neutral.
■ Neutral is balanced, and as such the most comfortable to skin, and the least likely to cause damage to spa equipment, and will allow hygiene agents to work optimally.

Alkaline
■ A low number of hydrogen ions make an alkaline pH.
■ An alkaline substance is defined as scoring between eight and fourteen on the pH scale.
■ A weakly alkaline substance is sea water with a pH of eight.
■ A strongly alkaline substance is bleach with a pH of fourteen.
■ Alkaline water can cause a hard scaly build-up which is destructive to spa equipment and can irritate skin.

Symptoms of chlorine or bromine poisoning

Chlorine or bromine poisoning is very rare, but very serious. Below are symptoms associated with the either toxic inhalation of chlorine gas, or other exposure to an excess of these chemicals.

Breathing trouble

Chlorine and bromine are gases and can damage airways and lungs, cause severe throat swelling and water to fill the lungs.

Vision and olfactory

Loss of vision and burning sensations of the eyes, nose, ears lips and tongue.

Gastrointestinal

Vomiting (or vomiting blood), abdominal pain and blood in the stool.

Skin

Burns appear alongside severe skin irritation.

Seeking help

In the case of suspected chlorine or bromine poisoning *seek medical help immediately* by calling the emergency services. Whilst you are waiting for aid:

1) Evacuate the area, and take any affected people into fresh air.
2) If chlorine is on skin or in eyes, wash with as much clean water as possible.

Testing the water

Water should be tested for both total alkalinity and pH, and can also be tested for other factors if contamination is suspected. Whilst the testing kits will be different depending on what you are assessing in the water, the manner of sampling will ely be the same.

- Wash your hands, as dirt or contaminants from your hands could affect test results.
- Use a clean plastic bottle rinsed through several times – avoid bringing glass into the spa area.
- Always sample from the same place every time. Keeping the stopper on the bottle, first rinse the outside three times in the water you are sampling from.

Chemicals such as chlorine and bromine used in keeping water hygienic are highly poisonous to all life forms. In very small quantities they will kill smaller bacteria without damaging human beings, but if ingested in larger amounts than at extremely low dilutions, it can cause illness or death.

Water testing should always be carried out whilst the pool is empty of bathers. Adjustments for pH or alkalinity can be hazardous and should take place in a spa area entirely free from clients with time allowed before re-entry is permitted.

4) Submerge the bottle around 30cm (12") under the water and fill to the level determined by your test kit (usually around 50ml mark).
5) Add your test tablet, shake the bottle vigorously, and check against the instructions of the test kit as to whether the water is the right colour.

Testing strips are also used to test water, and will come with their own instructions.

Total Alkalinity

Whilst the pH of the water is important, testing the Total Alkalinity or TA is actually a better indication. This is because the alkalinity of the water shows how able the water is to balance its own pH without intervention.

Measure and adjust (if necessary) the TA first, and adjusting the pH will often not be necessary.

pH levels

These can usually be easily adjusted with specialist spa products which will either increase or decrease the acidity of the water.

Ozone

The use of ultra violet ozone is becoming increasingly popular in spas as a way of avoiding harsh chemicals such as chlorine. Ozone is a natural way to kill bacteria and is far faster and more effective than chemicals. It also has other advantages such as reducing the side effects of chemicals such as red eyes, and also keeps water clearer. The expense of ozone generators, however, means they are a considered choice for spas. Ozone levels must be tested using electronic equipment.

Water-borne infections

As covered previously, water can present an environment in which germs and parasites can breed. Whilst proper hygiene and water monitoring is maintained this is unlikely to be a problem, but you should be aware of the main parasites and bacteria which could be present and cause problems.

Pseudomonas folliculitis

This is an infection of the hair follicles caused by the bacteria pseudomonas aeruginosa. Contamination will present itself as an inflamed rash of the follicles which will fade after a few days to a pigmented patch of skin. This pigment will disappear after another few weeks.

Fever and fatigue are occasionally reported as symptoms, but this is generally not a serious condition and will heal quickly without medical treatment. The spa water, however, must be tested and sanitised to remove the bacteria following any reports of this infection.

Avoiding contamination by pseudomonas aeruginosa is down to general good spa hygiene – regular water changes, a well-functioning filter and proper use of sanitiser.

Legionnaires' Disease

This is a bacterial infection which is contracted through inhaling water. For this reason spas and showers where water sprays out in a fine mist should be closely monitored. The disease is associated with poorly maintained water storage, and so water tanks and pipes should be well sealed and maintained to prevent infection.

Symptoms are very serious, resulting in potentially fatal pneumonia, and so legionnaires' disease should be considered as a significant hazard.

Respiratory and middle ear infections

A variety of bacteria and parasites can cause ear and respiratory problems. They are more likely to affect children, but can affect adult spa or pool users. Once again basic spa hygiene is the key to keeping these infections at bay – i.e. good filtration and water monitoring practices.

• KEY POINT

Illness can also be easily spread through warm water. Clients suffering from infections such as colds or stomach complaints should not use the spa area.

• KEY POINT

If shut down incorrectly, expensive equipment could be damaged, or the spa environment could even become hazardous. Always ensure you have proper training and help.

Water hygiene checklist

Problem	Possible Cause
Cloudy water	Filter problems
Skin irritation	pH or Total Alkalinity levels
Eye itching	Excess chlorine or low sanitiser levels
Algae or green growth	Low sanitiser levels
Excess foam and water line	Body oils and other contaminants
Oil on the water	Body oils, soap, dirt

Shut-down

Shutting down at the end of the day is a vital part of running a safe and well-maintained spa. A walk-through should be provided for individuals carrying out shut-down at closing time, but if one is not provided, ensure to ask for detailed instructions. If it is your first time shutting down the spa, you should be accompanied by a trained member of staff.

Turning off equipment will be a vital step, but equally important is to ensure certain aspects are still running if necessary. Keeping water clean and healthy for bathers is a round the clock process and should not be considered to have ceased merely because clients have left the spa.

Endpoints
By the end of this topic, you should understand:

■ basic water contamination safety
■ unique hygiene considerations of the spa area
■ the need for water testing and how you might carry out such tests
■ acid and alkaline balance, and the pH scale
■ chemicals or processes used to treat and sanitise water
■ possible parasites and diseases which could infect the spa area.

DON'T FORGET
TO LOGIN TO GAIN ACCESS TO YOUR **FREE** MULTI-MEDIA LEARNING RESOURCES

- ☐ **Over 40 minutes of instructional videos of all the key treatments**
- ☐ **Lesson plans and multiple choice and essay questions**
- ☐ **Interactive games and quizzes to help you to test your knowledge**

To login to use these resources visit
www.emspublishing.co.uk/spa and follow the onscreen instructions.

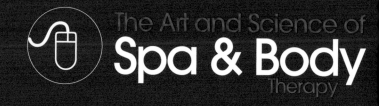

07

Hydrotherapy

The relaxing effect of water is widely known, and the use of water for treatments, or 'hydrotherapy' is extensively practised and widely enjoyed. Most therapists find this element offers very versatile procedures for a great range of clients. However, when using water safety is paramount.

Hydrotherapy has been used historically to treat disease, and whilst this is not the direct application in a modern treatment setting, there is some overlap. Using hot and cold water to gently stimulate the body the therapist can enact a number of health benefits as well as promoting relaxation.

TOPIC 1: WATER BASICS

As a therapist you'll need to know the different definitions of water types and the effect this can have on treatments. Many spas also pride themselves on the unique properties of their particular water.

WATER TYPES

Depending on which area of the country you are in or what style of hydrotherapy you are offering, the type of water used will vary.

Hard water

Hard water is sometimes seen as undesirable in the spa industry, because it has properties which make it less amenable to forming a lather from beauty products, and is also more likely to cause damage to the skin and equipment.

The reason for this is that hard water is so termed for its relatively high mineral content of calcium, magnesium and often other dissolved compounds. Hard and liquid soaps which usually lather in water, react to form a calcium or magnesium salt in the organic acid of the soap. So in very high concentrations of dissolved minerals it may not lather at all.

Additionally high temperatures can cause the calcium to react, making it adhere to metal. So in pipes which carry hot hard water, or other metals such as the element of a kettle or washing machine, a calcium scale can form which could eventually cause the unit to need replacing.

In a spa setting, however, hard water could be due to a healthy mineral content of natural spa water. In this case part of the therapy will involve exposure to these healthy minerals and can be seen as a desirable addition.

Hard water also has the benefit of washing soap substances from the skin more thoroughly giving a better 'clean' feeling.

Soft water

Soft water has little or no dissolved minerals in it and is derived from a source where elements such as calcium and magnesium are not present, such as peat or sandstone. It forms a generous lather with soap products, and does not form damaging

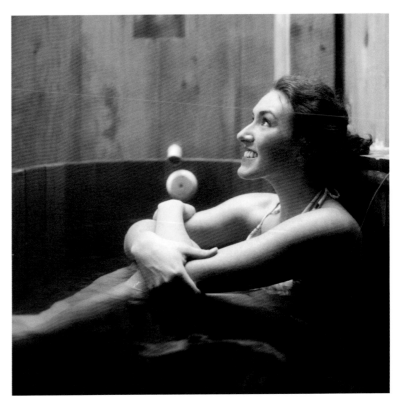

> **KEY POINT**
>
> Depending on the style of treatment you are offering and the area of the country you are in, the type of water you use can change considerably.

lime scale on hydrotherapy equipment. Excessive products however, may be difficult to rinse away in soft water, so manufacturer's directions must be strictly adhered to for foam baths etc when using this type of water.

This refers to salt-free water, such as filtered water, or water from a stream or natural spring source.

Water of this kind from unpolluted sources is in high demand as bottled drinking water, and so is not usually used in hydrotherapy treatments, although some high-end salons use filtered water to wash hair.

Fresh tap water, however, is often used for hydrotherapy treatments.

Salt water

Certain specialist treatment centres use seawater as a unique selling point for a particular spa. Notably these include thallasotherapy centres in Tunisia and Greece which claim that the local seawater has health qualities not found elsewhere.

WATER TEMPERATURE

Both very warm and very cool water can be used to therapeutic effect, but therapists should be well aware of potential hazards of extremes of temperature.

Cold water

Temperature can dip to freezing (0C) without damage to skin, and therapists are unlikely to have access to equipment which can bring liquids cooler than this. However, very low temperatures will come as an extreme shock to the client's central nervous system, which will react as if to a stress response. In very rare circumstances if this reaction is severe, then vulnerable clients such as older clients may be at risk of adverse shock symptoms such as seizure or heart attack.

For this reason hydrotherapy treatments which involve very cool water should never immerse or shower the head, for example plunge pools although nowadays the use of a swimming pool which is warmer is encouraged.

Hot water

As most therapists are well aware, over heated water can not only cause discomfort, but also burns. For this reason the utmost caution is necessary when using hydrotherapy treatments which call for heated water.

Before administering any treatment using heated water always check the water temperature on yourself first by running it over the inside of your wrist. In the case of baths, dip your elbow into the water first.

Having ascertained the water is comfortable for yourself, always check the temperature verbally with a client as you start treatment, and if necessary during treatment.

Never assume that because you have tested the water temperature of a piece of equipment previously that the temperature is still safe. Check every time you administer treatment.

● DID YOU KNOW?

Most tap water is treated with fluoride to protect the teeth. This is a very effective way to prevent tooth decay, but as fluoride is a disinfectant some people feel that bottled water is healthier to drink.

● KEY POINT

Water temperature should never drop below 45F or 7C. This is around the temperature of the average refrigerator, and is cool enough to stimulate the skin.

● KEY POINT

Check the water temperature every time for heated water treatments – even if you have checked it previously.

Effects of hot and cold water

Cold water	Hot water
Vasoconstriction	Vasodilatation
Skin pales (but can also flush slightly)	Skin flushes
Respiratory rate increases	Increase in oxygen consumption and metabolic rate
Skin and muscle tone improves (muscles tense)	Circulation increases, muscular relaxation
Internal body temperature increases, stimulating vital organs	Blood pressure decreases
Pulse rate increases	
Blood pressure increases	Body pH becomes more alkaline

On ceasing contact with water the basic effect for either hot or cold water is a balancing and ultimately relaxing sensation.

Respiratory rate drops

- Blood pressure and heart rate return to slightly lower than normal.
- Muscles relax.
- Sensation of well being often reported.

Endpoints
By the end of this topic, you should understand:

- the difference between hard and soft water
- hard and soft applications to the professional treatment setting
- various water-types used in treatment such as salt and freshwater and their possible applications
- the application of hot and cold water to create various health benefits in the body
- the physiological effects and variations of hot and cold.

TOPIC 2:
KNEIPP TREATMENT

Kneipp is a term which lends its name to many hydrotherapy treatments, and hails from a nineteenth century Bavarian monk, Sebastian Kneipp, who had a strong belief in the power of water to heal the body and eliminate toxins.

Treatment using Kneipp techniques is holistic in principle, which means that the practitioners should aim to involve all five senses as far as possible. The core procedures team hot and cold showers with rinses, baths and hot and cold compresses. At a more involved level, such as in a destination spa, nutritional therapy and treatments may be included as well as exercise treatments.

Principles of Kneipp

Many different hydrotherapy treatments have been developed around Kneipp principles, and the man himself liaised with many medical practitioners in order to develop a strong scientific basis for treatment.

Techniques were developed to address high and low blood pressure, circulation problems, and chronic conditions such as arthritis and rheumatism.

The principles understood to relate to Kniepp treatment include:

1) **Natural treatments.** Treatments often rely solely on the power of hot and cold water. However, where products are used, herbs, botanicals and natural oils form the key ingredients.
2) **Medical goals.** Kniepp designed his treatments for medical relief of chronic disorders, and treatments are strongly geared towards conditions such as circulatory problems, and joint pain.
3) **Increased immunity.** Kniepp principles are to invigorate the body and boost the natural immunity, conferring long term health benefits.
4) **Holistic.** Treatments are part of a wider focus

on diet and lifestyle. Where possible, treatment is part of a longer-term health plan.
5) **Use of nature.** Kniepp spas often take advantage of natural resources such as warm volcanic waters, and natural stones. Clients may walk barefoot over the smooth stones of a cool mountain stream, for example, as part of water stepping (see below).

A word on the history of Kniepp

Kniepp treatments originate from Germany, and original therapies involved using the cool waters of the River Danube to heal clients and deliver health benefits. The monk designed over 100 treatments using water in a variety of applications, and can be considered to a great extent to be the father of modern-day water hydrotherapy.

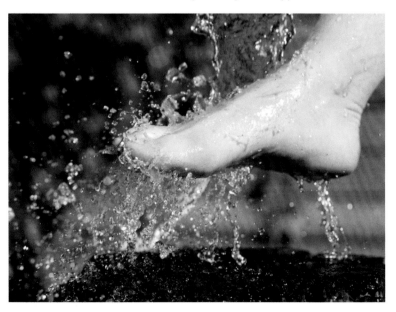

Kniepp's treatments included the use of water as:

- Ice
- Liquid
- Water vapour (steam).

Applications of these different forms of water include:

- Washing/rinsing
- Wraps
- Packs
- Compresses
- Poultices (hot)
- Affusions.

Using Kniepp can be as basic as applying cool and hot water, but for the comprehensive delivery of the principles behind the treatment the following should be adhered to:

1) **Hydrotherapy.** At the heart of Kniepp is the application of water for wellness. This means using hot and cold water to stimulate, energise and boost the health. The nervous system is toned and the immune system strengthened.

2) **Herbology.** Considered application of herbs to treat clients individually for a variety of health complaints. This method usually uses scientifically tested components to ensure the effectiveness of the herbs. Teas and foods are used in addition to herbs for the skin.

3) **Exercise.** Integral to many Kniepp hydrotherapy treatments is the application of gentle exercise. This is evident in treatments such as water stepping where the client enjoys cool water stimulation whilst maintaining a mild cardio work-out stepping in and out of the water.

4) **Nutrition.** As part of the herb treatment, nutrition is also attended to in classic Kniepp treatment. Ideally this means the use of a spa with a facility to provide healthy food for the client as they commence treatment. Focus for Kniepp is the use of fresh ingredients and raw vegetables.

5) **Harmonious lifestyle.** Living in harmony with the environment is a key principle of Kniepp and this can be the most elusive for a therapist to deliver. Many spas feature meditative practises and natural settings to achieve this aim. Ultimately the spa should provide a peaceful and attractive environment for their clients.

• KEY POINT

In essence Kniepp treatments are very simple. It is the skill of the therapist and the setting provided which adds a point of difference for the client.

• KEY POINT

Water stepping can be tiring even to clients who are physically fit, and extra care should be taken to avoid slippages. Always use a slip-guard, and remain at hand by the client's side in case they should stumble.

KNIEPP TREATMENTS

Kniepp treatments are very versatile, and can be performed in many different settings. The method behind treatment is the very basic application of hot and cold water, and so to an extent, how this is applied may vary with the spa or therapy setting. A salon, for example, might provide cool water application to the feet using a specialist bath or tub. Whilst a spa in a mountain setting could take advantage of a naturally occurring nearby stream to deliver the same treatment.

Water walking/stepping

Water walking or stepping is a fundamental Kniepp treatment, and one of the most widely used.

This treatment involves some exertion on the part of the client, and so can be regarded as a medical style of treatment rather than wholly for the purposes of relaxation.

It is an ideal circulation boosting exercise to be carried out early in the morning, or late evening to promote sleep.

1) Prior to treatment prepare a bathtub/footbath, or similar vessel with a slip-guard such as a rubber mat.

2) Fill the tub 12" deep (around 30cm) with cold water (around 45F).

3) The client wears a bathing costume for treatment and enters the tub with help if necessary.

4) Time the client as you direct them to walk in the water for two minutes raising the knees high, stepping in and out of the water with a stork-like gait using alternate feet.

5) After two minutes help the client to exit the water, and give them warm socks to put their feet in.

Hot and cold rinses

Hot and cold rinses can be performed in a bath or upright shower such as a Swiss shower. The body is doused in alternate hot and cold water for fifteen to twenty seconds at a time. This treatment can be performed using a Scotch hose, and may focus only on the knee to thigh area, or lower body.

Kniepp Bath

Kniepp baths team the soothing application of warm waters with specialist blends of natural herbs and oils. All five senses are exposed to:

1) **Touch.** The stimulating effect of the warm water. Clients can also be transferred from hot to cold baths to confer additional health benefits.
2) **Taste.** Water or herbal teas may be drunk before or after treatments.
3) **Sight.** Kniepp baths are often supplied with fresh petals floating on the surface to add a visual element to the treatment.
4) **Sound.** The soothing running of the water can be augmented with water-sounds in the background supplied naturally by the setting or using recorded music.
5) **Smell.** Intoxicating fragrances from the oils and herbs help the client relax fully into the treatment. Herbal remedies in the bath may confer nutritional benefits to the skin with vitamins and minerals absorbed from the treatment.

Kniepp bath application

Kniepp baths can be a full body treatment or applied to isolated body parts to deliver different benefits. The most usual delivery is full immersion, but in certain circumstances the therapist may want to consider these variations:

1) **Arm bath.** The arms only are immersed. This can be a useful treatment for a client not suited to more rigorous styles of Kniepp bath, as they can enjoy the benefits of hot and cold water on their arms only.
2) **Foot bath.** Ideal for clients with poor circulation in their lower body. The application of a foot bath provides a boost for those suffering from conditions such as varicose veins as it tones the vascular system. Cold feet can also be treated using this method.
3) **Hip bath.** A variation of the full Kniepp bath which immerses the hips only in varying hot and cold water, Suitable for clients for whom fuller bath methods might be too vigorous.
4) **Half bath.** As with the hip bath, but slightly more stimulatory, as it covers the hips, back, buttocks and feet.

5) **Three-quarter bath.** As above but more of the thigh is submerged.

A word on herbal additions

Kniepp herbs are a vital part of delivering an effective bath treatment. Popular additions include balm mint, chamomile, lavender, meadow flower and pine needle. Those interested in the use of herbs for therapeutic purposes can consider training to be a herbologist.

DELIVERING A KNIEPP BATH

1) Prepare the bath to the required temperature and add treatment powder or oil as required (see below for Kniepp bath types).
2) Check the bath temperature with your elbow.
3) Client wears swimwear/disposable underwear and is given a robe if they need to move to a different treatment area.
4) Assist the client into the bath, and check the water temperature is comfortable.
5) If necessary, place a cool damp cloth on the client's forehead. This is particularly effective for stimulating and detoxifying baths such as the Mustard Bath or Seaweed Bath.
6) Provide water or herbal tea as required.
7) Leave the client to relax for fifteen minutes.
8) Check on the client and re-supply water or herbal tea as required.
9) Depending on the length of bath (see manufacturer's instructions for treatment types) the client will most likely take from half an hour to an hour. Check every ten minutes for comfort and add more hot water if necessary.

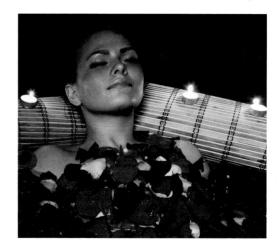

10) Follow treatment with a full half-hour rest wrapped in towels in a relaxation area where possible. Provide plenty of liquids.

11) Finish the treatment with a cold shower where applicable.

DIFFERENT TYPES OF KNIEPP BATH

Depending on the temperature and the herbs used, Kniepp baths can be delivered for a wide range of conditions.

Mud bath

Treats:

- Rheumatism
- Sciatica
- Neuritis (nerve inflammation)
- Lumbago (lower back pain)
- Joint pain.

Whey powder bath

Whey powder baths are otherwise known as milk baths. They have been used since ancient times to nourish the skin, and Cleopatra bathed in milk. These baths are sometimes called lacto-med-derm bath (from 'lacto' meaning 'from milk', 'med' from 'medical, and 'derm' for 'skin health').

Treats:

- Ageing dry skin
- Dermatitis
- Psoriasis
- Acne
- Eczema
- Sunburn.

Mustard powder bath

Mustard is well-known for its stimulatory qualities, and can be an excellent tonic for the lungs and respiratory system as well as the circulation in general. The mustard opens up pores and encourages sweating, whilst refreshing and soothing the skin with natural oils.

Treats:

- Fatigue
- Muscle soreness
- Muscle ache
- Insomnia.

• KEY POINT

Mud treatments are sometimes known as fango mud treatments. Fango simply refers to mud of a volcanic origin. Other mud can come from peat bogs, sea-beds, or various mineral-rich sources.

This is famous for delivering rich skin-nourishing qualities. Mud baths are supplied in powdered form and can be easily added to warm water.

Seaweed powder bath

Seaweed is flash-frozen to ensure the full nourishing skin effects are maintained. As a powder it is then added to bath water where it re-hydrates, conferring many mineral qualities such as iodine vitamins and enzymes. As with seaweed wraps (see Chapter 8: Body masks and wraps) the seaweed is also a detoxifying agent for the body.

Some seaweed treatments are fragranced, but ideally the natural seaweed aroma should be maintained as this is part of the Kniepp principle of delivering full holistic treatment.

Treats:

- Cellulite
- Poor circulation
- Skin tone
- Detoxification requirements.

Essential oils bath

This is one of the most common baths used in spas as it provides a highly indulgent and relaxing treatment experience. Scented oils to suit the clients preference are added to the bath for deep relaxation and muscle soothing. Petals are also often added for visual purposes.

Treats:

- Stress
- Fatigue
- Muscle pain
- Tension.

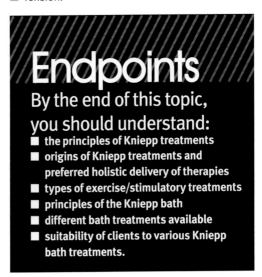

Endpoints

By the end of this topic, you should understand:

- the principles of Kniepp treatments
- origins of Kniepp treatments and preferred holistic delivery of therapies
- types of exercise/stimulatory treatments
- principles of the Kniepp bath
- different bath treatments available
- suitability of clients to various Kniepp bath treatments.

TOPIC 3:
UNIQUE PROPERTIES OF HYDROTHERAPY

Water or hydrotherapy can create a diverse and unique range of treatments. Due to the gentle nature of these treatments and the supportive nature of water, it is also very well suited to a range of client types.

THERAPEUTIC PROPERTIES OF WATER

People have indulged in the therapeutic and sensory properties of water for as far back in history as has been recorded. Spas as we know them today were originally founded on the principles of healing water, and this concept has remained in place for many modern treatments.

BENEFITS OF HYDROTHERAPY

Hydrotherapy comes with a diverse list of benefits which you will find very useful as a therapist.

Range of client types

Depending on the hydrotherapy used, many treatments are practical for clients who may otherwise be unable to regularly enjoy relaxing treatments. These include clients who are very overweight, as well as those with restricted mobility and physical disabilities.

Improvement of cardiovascular health

Contact with warm water helps tone and improve cardiovascular health, stimulating dilation of capillaries, and improving detoxification.

Muscle relaxation

Support in water instantly relaxes and supports muscles, as well as soothing joint and other pain.

Temperature control

As water can be employed to surround the body and set to various temperatures it offers therapists

● DID YOU KNOW?

As a basic element this simple compound of hydrogen and oxygen has many unique qualities which make it essential for life on the planet, and it accounts for 50-70% of the human body. Some even theorise that human beings have evolved from water-based life-forms.

a uniquely accurate method of employing heat treatment and all the associated benefits.

Buoyancy

The buoyancy of the human body in water is a key aspect of many hydrotherapy treatments, and in particular flotation tank therapy. As it floats the body becomes weightless, aiding relaxation of the muscles. Adipose tissue, or fat, is less dense than muscle and floats well, so increased adipose tissue will help buoyancy.

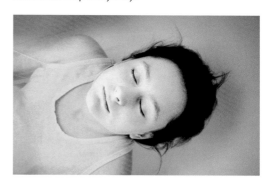

A word on buoyancy

Buoyancy is achieved when the floating subject is less dense than the water below. For this reason buoyancy is enhanced over a wide surface area, as this lessens the density of any one point of the object over a given volume of water. It is for this reason that if you stand in water you will sink to the bottom, but laying on your back can cause you to float.

Water hygiene

Water hygiene is extremely important, and therapists should be aware that this element can be an easy conduit of infections and disease as well as bacterial growth. For this reason water used in a professional spa setting is subject to various tests and hygiene treatments to protect clients from infection and illness. Water-borne infections and water-testing is covered in more detail in Chapter 6: Spas.

Effect of water on the skin

Prolonged exposure to water can cause wrinkling or 'pruning' of the skin on the fingertips and toes.

Endpoints

By the end of this topic, you should understand:

- the suitability of water as a therapeutic treatment
- a brief history of hydrotherapy
- issues unique to water-therapy such as buoyancy and muscle soothing
- water hygiene issues
- the effect of water on the skin.

TOPIC 4: FLOTATION THERAPY

As the name suggests, flotation allows the client to lie suspended in water, completely relaxed with no part of their body in hard contact with a solid surface. Many people find this experience very peaceful and soothing.

History of flotation

This treatment became popular in the UK in the last few decades with the invention of specialised flotation tanks. Prior to this flotation as a form of relaxation has been widely used in the natural setting of the Dead Sea.

Flotation tanks were actually designed in the USA as early as the 1950s by scientists looking to experiment with the effects of 'total sensory deprivation'. In pursuit of this end Dr John Lilly – a neuroscientist at the National Institute of Mental Health in Maryland – invented a darkened tank in which subjects could lie weightless with no sights or sounds of the outside world. The initial design was to explore and experiment on the idea of consciousness and how it related to brain function. The theory was that if all stimuli were deprived the notion of how the mind regards itself without relating to the outside world could be explored with better accuracy.

The main result, however, was that the scientists discovered an environment which was completely relaxing for subjects, and the flotation tank went on to gain popularity for this purpose in the US.

THE SCIENCE OF FLOTATION

Normal water – even salty seawater – is less dense than the human body. This means when you swim or bathe in this water you will naturally sink to the bottom. Flotation therapy, however, uses a natural phenomenon which occurs in the Dead Sea in a therapeutic setting. Water is saturated with salt, changing the density of the water and causing a person to float rather than sink.

The Dead Sea has been a tourist spot since the first century. This ancient attraction was once an actual ocean, but became landlocked due to natural drifting of continents. As the sea was cut off in a hot area with low humidity, a great deal of water evaporated, leaving highly salted water behind. The result was a 'dead' sea in which the salt concentration meant people could float naturally, but no species of marine life could survive.

THE FLOTATION TANK

Flotation tanks are widely available and relatively inexpensive for therapeutic purposes. They do, however require a reasonable amount of space, and should preferably be located in a very quiet areas – although earplugs can be provided.

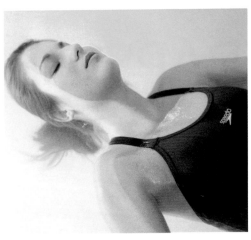

Nirvana Spa - www.nirvanaspa.co.uk

The tank is filled with ten inches (around 25cm) of water, which due to its high salt content is enough for any individual to float free of the bottom of the tank. A lid is closed on the individual, and depending on personal preference, the lights can be turned out to create total darkness.

Tanks come in different shapes, with egg-shaped being a more popular modern design. Additional features could include:

A canopy (rather than a lid)

Two-way speakers for client ease of mind whilst floating (allowing them to communicate with the

When speaking with clients 'sensory deprivation' may sound intimidating, so ensure you talk around the term and explain all its benefits.

therapist if need be), or to play relaxing music.

Non-drip ceilings to prevent salt water raining into the eyes.

The density of the salted water is achieved by around 31% salt content, which can be achieved by adding either Epsom salts or Dead Sea salts. There is some debate between the two, as Dead Sea salts are thought to give a better sensation of weightlessness, but Epsom salts confer mineral properties to the skin, such as detoxification.

Principles of flotation therapy

Whilst flotation tanks are no longer known as sensory deprivation chambers, the fundamentals of this early design are still very much part of the experience. Today, floatation rooms are more widely used where more than one client shares the experience in a small room taken up entirely by a small pool of water. The environment may be enhanced by the use of piped music and candles or soft lighting. These rooms should be situated in a quiet areas of the spa. The major benefits of flotation are achieved by ensuring the basic principles are met to give the client a sensation, which as far as possible feels like floating on air.

1) **Weightlessness.** This is achieved by the salt content which allows the entire body to float as if weightless.
2) **Lessened skin sensation.** Water is heated to skin temperature which gives the sensation of removing physical body boundaries.
3) **Sound and vision.** Ear-plugs can be used and lights turned out, although neither is essential for relaxation if the client feels uncomfortable.
4) Thought to be the equivalent of a good nights sleep.

BENEFITS OF FLOTATION THERAPY
1) Muscle relaxation

Even at rest muscles are in constant activity, and floating weightless enables them to completely relax in every part of the body. This is also thought to help aid injury recovery time.

2) Meditation

A float is normally recommended for between twenty to sixty minutes. After forty minutes of flotation the brain enters the theta brainwave

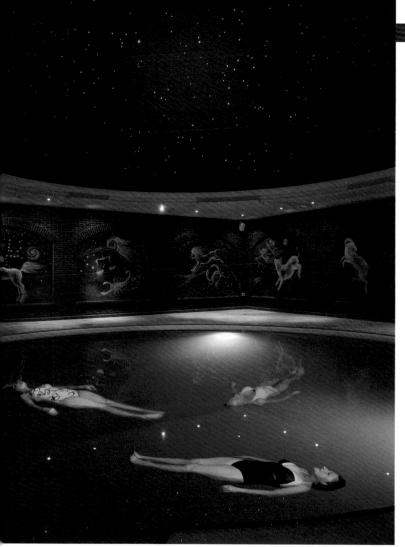

Nirvana Spa - www.nirvanaspa.co.uk

small spaces. Clients actively suffering from this condition are unlikely to volunteer for treatment, but many people have a mild version and are averse to the darkened or soundless aspect of the flotation experience. In this circumstance clients can be reassured that the lights can be left on, and they are free to leave the tank at any time of their own accord. Claustrophobia can be overcome in many cases by using a flotation room rather than a tank.

Other contraindications

- Open wounds or cuts – these may react painfully to the salt content of the water.
- Contact lens wearers – lenses should be removed before treatment.
- Fungal infections.
- Viral infections.
- Skin diseases.
- Ear infections or problems.
- Fever, diarrhoea or similar illness.
- Any other condition under medical supervision of which you are unsure.

state which is associated with deep relaxation, meditation and later sleep stages. Many clients remain conscious in this stage, and report heightened creativity and problem solving abilities, whilst others enjoy a deep and restful sleep.

3) Skin health

The mineral content of the Epsom salts (if used) confer skin softening qualities.

CONTRAINDICATIONS

Flotation is a very gentle therapy, and there are few major contraindications. Therapists should, however, be aware of some possible conditions which could affect treatment.

Claustrophobia

The main contraindication which therapists are likely to come across is claustrophobia – a fear of

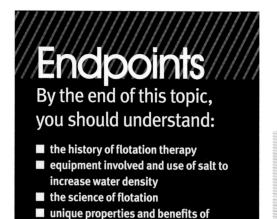

Endpoints
By the end of this topic, you should understand:

- the history of flotation therapy
- equipment involved and use of salt to increase water density
- the science of flotation
- unique properties and benefits of flotation therapy
- contraindications and treatment restrictions for flotation therapy.

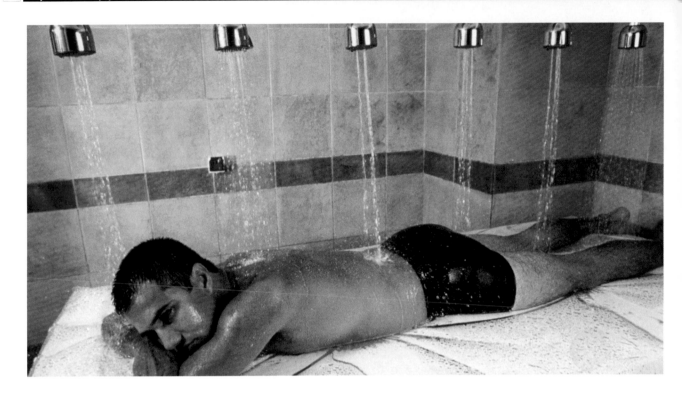

TOPIC 5:
AFFUSION SHOWERS

This is a highly versatile type of shower which is designed to rain water from numerous shower heads. The client lies horizontal whilst this takes place in a specially designed bed and room for the purpose of water-therapy.

SHOWER DESIGN

Affusion showers come in different makes and models, with the most modern incorporating a wet-bed beneath an integrated overhanging unit of five shower heads. Different styles may also be comprised of a single metal rail of shower heads which plumbs into a unit in the wall, and can hang over a therapist's choice of couch.

HISTORY OF THE AFFUSION SHOWER

Affusion showers are named after the religious practice of baptism, and stems from the Latin word meaning to 'pour over'. In the more modern sense they were originally used for the purposes of

• KEY POINT

Affusion showers are most commonly used in conjunction with other treatments, and are a particularly luxurious way of rinsing away body wraps and masks (see Chapter 8: Body masks and wraps).

cardiovascular health in the setting of Swiss health spas – hence they are sometimes known as 'Swiss showers'. Although in spa therapy practice this term in fact relates to a slightly different type of shower (Topic 6: Swiss showers).

The stimulating effect of water on the circulation can be greatly enhanced by temperature control, allowing alternatively hot and cold water to rain down on the skin. This boosts the activity of the vascular system, toning and strengthening body tissues.

For spa treatments, however, affusion showers are generally used to relax, and so temperatures are set to emit a constant soothing warmth.

BENEFITS OF THE AFFUSION SHOWER

Affusion showers can be a wonderful way to offer the gentle soothing benefits of changing water temperature. They have many benefits, in particular for less mobile clients.

1) **Circulation health.** Affusion showers are excellent for stimulating circulation, as they apply light yet constant pressure to the vasculature, toning and conditioning. For this reason they can also help the flow of lymph through the body, which also aids detoxification. Clients may also find a benefit to areas of the body with sluggish circulation meaning an improvement to conditions such as poor circulation and cellulite.

2) **Heat.** The warmth of the water on the client's body provides instant heat and relaxation of the muscles. Teamed with the massaging effect of the water this greatly enhances the ability of the therapist to massage areas of deep tension more effectively and relax the muscles fibres.

3) **Massage.** The constant soothing effect of water raining down on the body creates a massage effect which can be varied in pressure according to the capabilities of the equipment. Rather than being used as a massage in its own right, however, affusion showers are often used in combination with manual massage from a therapist.

A word on massage in affusion showers

Massage techniques are covered in more detail in Chapter 9: Massage techniques. However, affusion showers should be accompanied by massage. This means that the client remains completely immobile, and no limbs are moved as in certain styles. This means the following massage styles are not suited to affusion showers:

■ *Thai massage.*

■ *Sports massage which use deep tissue techniques that are not suited to affusion showers.*

Instead the massage should be of a style which incorpoates long effleurage strokes to soothe the body, aid circulation, and stimulate the clearance and movement of the lymphatic system.

DELIVERY OF AFFUSION SHOWERS

Affusion showers can be modified to suit a vast number of client requirements and treatments. The following is a basic procedure for delivery of affusion showers prior to further treatment such as massage.

1) The client is directed to change into suitable swimwear or disposable underwear.

2) Robes should be provided if the client needs to move to different treatment areas. Welcome the client into the treatment room and talk them briefly through the process.

3) Direct the client to lie face down on the couch.

4) Start the shower, and check with the client that the water temperature is comfortable.

5) Leave the client to relax alone under the shower.

6) If administering massage during the shower treatment, return after five minutes to begin manual massage.

Endpoints

By the end of this topic, you should understand:

■ **the different uses of affusion showers in addition to a standalone treatment**

■ **equipment and set-up of a range of affusion showers**

■ **history of the affusion shower**

■ **benefits of the affusion shower**

■ **how to deliver a standard affusion shower treatment.**

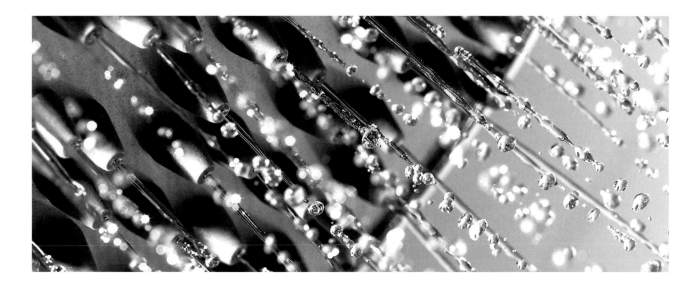

TOPIC 6:
SWISS SHOWER

This is another version of the affusion shower, and is sometimes referred to by the latter name. The difference as usually understood in the spa industry, however, is that whilst the affusion shower is delivered to a client lying horizontally on a couch, the Swiss shower treatment is received vertically. For this reason the Swiss shower is often employed as a more stimulating and invigorating version of the horizontal affusion shower.

EQUIPMENT

Swiss shower cabinet/jets

The Swiss shower comprises several vertically set rows of shower heads, which can number from five to over fifteen. Unlike the affusion shower where the power of gravity allows water to gently spray onto the body, the Swiss shower uses high power pumps, which surge water out in high powered but slim 'needle-spray' jets.

Swiss showers may be built into a cubicle, very similar in appearance to a domestic shower, or built into a tiled alcove. Stand-alone Swiss showers can be plumbed into the floor of any tiled area, and consist of a square metal frame reaching to shoulder height, within which the powerful jets can spray water inwards.

A word about Swiss showers

High water-pressure for Swiss showers is essential for effective treatment. However, pressure which is too firm can feel uncomfortable and even bruise the skin. Check the pressure of the water yourself using the inside of your arm, before the client enters.

PRINCIPLES OF SWISS SHOWER

The Swiss shower teams water massage with varying water temperature. So the client alternatively experiences warm and cold water on the skin alongside pressure sensations. This has the dual advantages of both extremes of water temperature, from a cool 45F to warm/hot 105F

BENEFITS OF SWISS SHOWER

1) Warm water/cold water stimulation

As described earlier in this chapter, both warm and cool water have an effect on the body which in the short term and controlled setting of a treatment are very beneficial.

Cold water acts to tone the muscular and vascular systems, increasing pulse rate as the body works to draw blood to the internal organs and keep warm.

Warm water also stimulates the metabolism and respiratory system, driving blood back into the skin and away from the vital organs, and flushing out toxins as it does so. The managed application of both extremes of temperature works as a tonic for the body, and combined with vigorous massage works as a tonic for the entire system.

2) Relaxation

Following treatment the nervous system returns to normal and the muscles enter a state of deep relaxation. Having maintained a state of muscle tone during cold water therapy and increased blood flow from temperature changes, tension in the muscles will be soothed, and conditions involving joint pain such as arthritis often also benefit.

3) Cardiovascular health

As long as temperatures remain within the correct spectrum, treatment acts as a mild cardiovascular work-out for the body, and can be particularly useful for clients who are unable to exercise for other reasons.

4) After scrubs/masks/wraps

Swiss showers can act as a stimulating way to remove body masks after a mask or wrap treatment (see Chapter 8: Body masks and wraps). Whilst affusion showers can also be used for this purpose, the higher pressure and vertical position of Swiss showers can remove products more effectively.

Scotch hoses can be used in conjunction with many different hydrotherapy treatments, but are most commonly used with Swiss shower treatments. They consist of a powerful handheld

• KEY POINT

Like the affusion shower, the Swiss shower can be adapted to many different treatment ends, both proceeding, preceding, or as a standalone treatment.

• KEY POINT

Scotch hoses are often an addition to Swiss shower treatments, as they enhance the effects of the water pressure.

unit through which the therapist can direct high pressure jets of water to the client's body as they enjoy the stimulating effect of the Swiss shower. The handheld hose is usually part of a wall mounted unit with options to vary pressure and heat.

Benefits of Scotch Hose

1) **Delivers additional massage.** Clients can enjoy an additional massage alongside their Swiss shower.

2) **Targeted massage.** Stronger massage can be directed to known points of tension. Therapists with knowledge of acupressure points can also use this piece of equipment for this purpose in a hydrotherapy setting.

3) **Alternative temperature.** Scotch hose can be used to deliver a contrasting temperature to the Swiss shower (i.e. cold Scotch hose when the Swiss shower is hot or vice versa) increasing the effectiveness of the hot/cold stimulatory effect.

4) **Rinsing of masks or products.** The hose can be directed to rinse product from areas where it can be hard to remove such as the backs of knees or inside of elbows.

Endpoints
By the end of this topic, you should understand:

- the difference between Swiss showers and affusion showers
- uses of the Swiss shower in a therapy setting
- likely set-up/equipment for the Swiss shower
- benefits of Swiss shower therapy
- scotch hose as an addition to Swiss shower treatment.

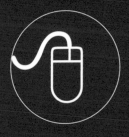

DON'T FORGET
TO LOGIN TO GAIN ACCESS TO YOUR **FREE** MULTI-MEDIA LEARNING RESOURCES

- ☐ **Over 40 minutes of instructional videos of all the key treatments**
- ☐ **Lesson plans and multiple choice and essay questions**
- ☐ **Interactive games and quizzes to help you to test your knowledge**

To login to use these resources visit
www.emspublishing.co.uk/spa and follow the onscreen instructions.

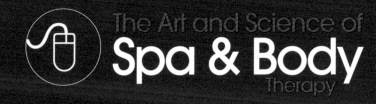

The Art and Science of
Spa & Body
Therapy

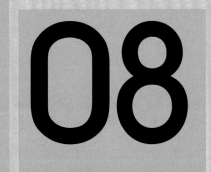

Body masks and wraps

Masks can be applied to the body to enact many beneficial effects such as hydration and detoxification. Body wraps are a relaxing and indulgent way to activate body masks, and are readily combined with other treatments such as exfoliation and massage. Wraps are also a useful way to add heat to a treatment and stimulate perspiration and detoxification. For this reason wraps have also been developed for inch-loss purposes and are used with agents such as mud and seaweed.

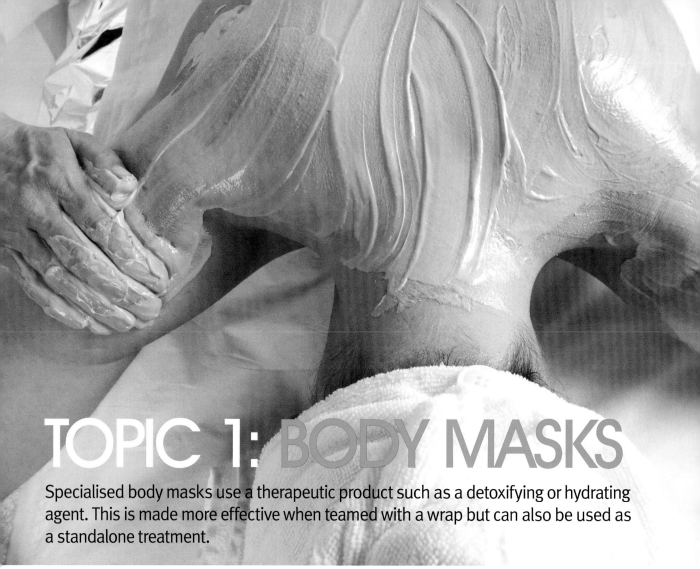

TOPIC 1: BODY MASKS

Specialised body masks use a therapeutic product such as a detoxifying or hydrating agent. This is made more effective when teamed with a wrap but can also be used as a standalone treatment.

● DID YOU KNOW?

Body masks are a common feature of spa 'rituals' where the client enjoys several treatments in a day or half-day session.

Types of body mask

Body masks consist of a thick medium which is applied directly onto the client's skin. Depending on the effect required by the client the mask ingredients may vary. They may include moisturising elements such as essential oils, detoxifying components such as seaweed, or a number of other specialised additions.

ANTI-CELLULITE MASK

Many clients seek treatment for cellulite, which can be alleviated rather than cured, by therapeutic detoxifying treatments. Cellulite is thought to consist of toxins which have become trapped in between the fat cells, particularly on the hip and thighs in women. Stimulating the body's natural detoxification pathways should substantially improve the elimination process thereby improving the appearance and tone of the skin.

These treatments rely on specially developed products which may consist of one or more of the following ingredients:

- ■ **Detoxifying mud**
- ■ **Moisturising/stimulating essential oils**
- ■ **Cellulite specific gels.**

These are often combined for maximum effect, and depending on the active ingredient for the specific treatment of cellulite will vary in price. Products manufactured by high-end beauty companies will naturally tend to command premium rates, but these products also have the conviction of science behind them.

Current favourite product additions for the active treatment of cellulite include:

1) **Caffeine.**
2) **Aminophylline** – a bronchiole dilator also found in skin creams which is thought to be able to dilate capillaries when applied to the skin.

3) **Lemon oil** – a historic treatment for cellulite with added antibacterial qualities.

4) **Retinol** – the active form of vitamin A. Vitamin A is thought to play a part in skin repair when taken orally. Retinol is thought to confer similar benefits when applied topically.

5) **L-Carnitine** – this stimulatory enzyme is said to increase the body's metabolic rate as well as reduce the capacity for cells to store fats.

6) **Herbal extracts** - many herbal extracts help in detoxification with favourites including juniper and rosemary.

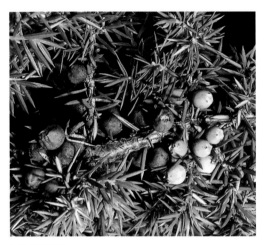

Juniper berries

7) **Vitamin E and C** – both of these ingredients help strengthen skin, aid repair and stimulate collagen synthesis.

8) **Algae** – see 'seaweed masks' for more information later in this chapter.

HERBAL MASKS

Herbal masks are distinct from those which use herbs as a single part of their active ingredients such as anti-cellulite masks. Instead they use only herbs and call upon specialised equipment to infuse bandages and linen.

In mask treatments the herbs used are often designed to induce perspiration. These include:

- **Rosemary**
- **Peppermint**
- **Lavender**
- **Cypress**
- **Juniper.**

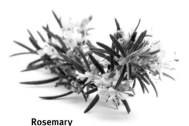

Rosemary

Additional equipment for herb masks
Moist heat unit

In order to deliver a herbal mask the therapist must have access to a moist heat unit. This is a small stainless steel tank which can hold heated water. Herbs are infused into the water in much the same way as tea from tea-bags, but on a large scale. The device then holds the bandages or linens at the correct temperature ready for treatment.

Packages of therapeutic herbs

These are specialist bags of therapeutic herbs designed and manufactured for use in the moist-heat unit. They come in various formulations and incorporate different blends of herbs.

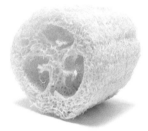

MOISTURISING MASKS

In order for moisturising products to be better absorbed by the body professional exfoliation is imperative for this treatment. Favoured methods include dry body brushing or moist loofah exfoliation. This enables the skin to fully benefit from the moisturising effect, removing dead skin cells and stimulating circulation.

Special attention should also be paid to moisturising dry areas of the body, which are usually:

- **Elbows**
- **Kneecaps**
- **Feet.**

Ingredients for moisturising wraps can vary, and will often take the form of products already favoured by the salon for other treatments such as facials. These ensure a high quality moisturising agent is delivered to the skin. Fragrances such as rose may be added for the dual purpose of hydration and relaxation, but generally the contents of a moisturising mask will be very diverse. Soothing moisturising serum followed by dry skin oil and concluded with a rich body butter is a standard combination.

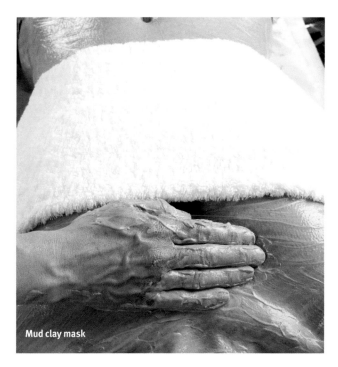

Mud clay mask

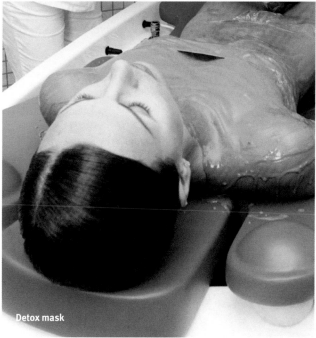

Detox mask

MUD/CLAY MASK

Mud or clay masks are commonly used for drawing out interstitial fluid, as well as generating inch and weight loss.

Wet mud or clay is painted onto the skin either using gloved hands, or preferably painted on in smooth strokes with a wide brush. As the clay or mud dries it draws out impurities and fluids from the skin, creating manually induced perspiration. The result is that the skin is firmer and clearer.

Clay mask mineral properties

Many kinds of different clay and mud can be used, and spas in particular often have access to locations of high mineral content. For this reason any special mud or clay treatment should be emphasised to clients for superior skin-nourishing content.

Mud and clay packs can include:

1) **Organic volcanic ash.**
2) **Peat from bogs.**
3) **Mineral sea mud.**
4) **Clay from mineral-rich areas.**

All are usually available as a powder which the therapist can mix ready for their client.

● **DID YOU KNOW?**

As part of a spa ritual, clients may be offered additional treatments for example a foot massage or a head massage to complement the mask/ wrap treatment.

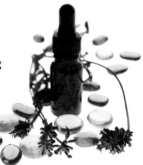

DETOX MASK

Detox body masks can sometimes fall under the category of seaweed or herbal wraps, but they may also use their own specific detoxifying ingredients. Similarly, they may or may not be designed to induce inch loss.

Because detox masks are designed to induce perspiration they are always used in conjunction with a wrap. Depending on the style of wrap used (bandage or body) the wrap may cause fluid loss which is measurable by a tape-measure. Whichever method is used, however, perspiration will occur and a degree of fluid-loss will take place.

Ingredients used in detox masks are those associated with stimulation and are circulation boosting. Popular oils and botanicals include:

1) **Citrus (gels or oils) –**
   lemon, orange, grapefruit.
2) **Rosemary.**
3) **Juniper berry.**
4) **Cypress.**

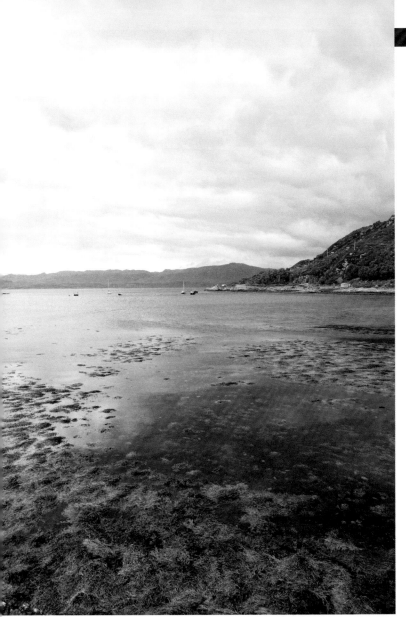

Skin nourishing

Seaweed is thought to nourish the skin by conferring a wide spectrum of minerals and vitamins directly to the epidermis. Seaweed masks are comprised of algae and seaweed specifically chosen for their detoxifying and skin nourishing properties.

Mineral content

Seaweed is unparalleled in its natural mineral composition, and contains:

- **Vitamin A**
- **B Vitamins (B1, B2, B6, B12)**
- **Vitamin C**
- **Vitamin E**
- **Vitamins K**
- **Copper**
- **Iron**
- **Potassium**
- **Zinc**
- **Iodine.**

Many of these minerals help break down the body's fatty deposits, which in turn helps stimulate the removal and metabolism of the toxins which cause cellulite. Additionally, the vitamins in particular are thought to work as emollients (skin softeners).

Seaweed masks also contain other hydrating and therapeutic ingredients, which are blended with an activator. Additionally, collagen can be added for a particularly luxurious mask with age-defying properties, but this combination is expensive and usually reserved for face masks only.

SEAWEED MASK

Seaweed masks have become popular for a number of reasons, but are generally upheld as excellent detoxifying agents. Seaweed is also associated with inch-loss style wraps which induce weight loss. They also stimulate circulation as part of their detoxifying abilities.

The advantages most often cited for seaweed masks include:

Cellulite

Seaweed masks are the key ingredient used in tackling cellulite in the skin. The mineral content of the masks, combined with their detoxifying abilities is thought to make them the most effective for this purpose.

• KEY POINT

Seafood or shellfish allergy can act as an important contraindication for seaweed wraps.

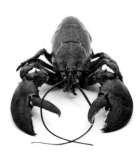

A word about seaweed odour

Seaweed can smell quite strongly of the sea, and whilst this helps therapists know the provenance and quality of their products the fragrance is not as popular with clients. For this reason many manufacturers use perfumes to mask the seaweed smell. These can be natural botanical oils or manufactured fragrance. If possible select masks which opt for natural ingredients only.

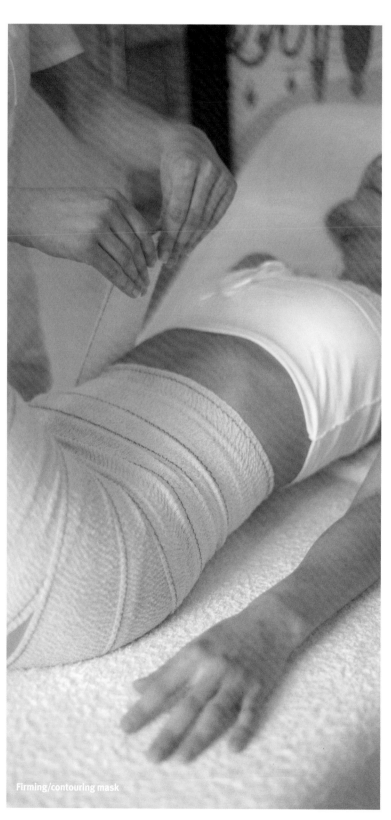

Firming/contouring mask

FIRMING/CONTOURING MASK

Firming and contouring treatments are a further popular way to utilise the qualities of wrap treatments, and like detoxification masks are always used in conjunction with a wrap.

Contouring masks are usually specifically designed for weight loss purposes, and utilise a specialised bandage style of wrapping material (see Topic 3: Different wrap m ethods). As this method wraps right around the limbs Egyptian mummy style it is able to enact more efficient drawing out of toxins and interstitial fluids, leading to inch loss.

With a contouring wrap designed specifically for inch loss it is necessary to measure the client before and after treatment in order for them to recognise the areas of their body where the wrap has been effective. As wraps of this kind genuinely deliver inch loss, most clients are delighted with this aspect of the treatment.

A word on contouring wraps

Contouring wraps deliver inch loss mainly by draining excess interstitial fluid from cells. This is excess fluid which would normally be naturally drained away by the lymphatic system. If the body is overloaded with toxins this system can become sluggish so contouring wraps can remove the excess. Whilst inch loss is attained using this method, however, it is not the same as weight loss. Body fat as measured on an electronic scale will remain the same or may even seem proportionally higher in relation to water loss. For this reason clients should be encouraged to drink plenty of water to re-hydrate their body and speed up toxin removal.

Areas of the body to measure for inch loss

Most therapists use a standard tape measure, as this is the easiest tool and readily understood by clients. Callipers as described in Chapter 2 are not an appropriate tool for this purpose.

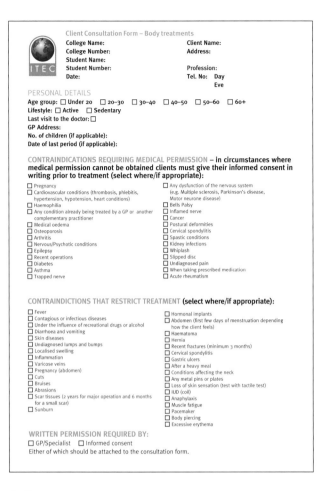

Client Consultation Form – Body treatments

College Name:
College Number:
Student Name:
Student Number:
Date:

Client Name:
Address:

Profession:
Tel. No: Day
Eve

PERSONAL DETAILS

Age group: ☐ Under 20   ☐ 20–30   ☐ 30–40   ☐ 40–50   ☐ 50–60   ☐ 60+
Lifestyle: ☐ Active   ☐ Sedentary
Last visit to the doctor: ☐
GP Address:
No. of children (if applicable):
Date of last period (if applicable):

CONTRAINDICATIONS REQUIRING MEDICAL PERMISSION – **in circumstances where medical permission cannot be obtained clients must give their informed consent in writing prior to treatment (select where/if appropriate):**

☐ Pregnancy
☐ Cardiovascular conditions (thrombosis, phlebitis, hypertension, hypotension, heart conditions)
☐ Haemophilia
☐ Any condition already being treated by a GP or another complementary practitioner
☐ Medical oedema
☐ Osteoporosis
☐ Arthritis
☐ Nervous/Psychotic conditions
☐ Epilepsy
☐ Recent operations
☐ Diabetes
☐ Asthma
☐ Trapped nerve

☐ Any dysfunction of the nervous system (e.g. Multiple sclerosis, Parkinson's disease, Motor neurone disease)
☐ Bells Palsy
☐ Inflamed nerve
☐ Cancer
☐ Postural deformities
☐ Cervical spondylitis
☐ Spastic conditions
☐ Kidney infections
☐ Whiplash
☐ Slipped disc
☐ Undiagnosed pain
☐ When taking prescribed medication
☐ Acute rheumatism

CONTRAINDICTIONS THAT RESTRICT TREATMENT **(select where/if appropriate):**

☐ Fever
☐ Contagious or infectious diseases
☐ Under the influence of recreational drugs or alcohol
☐ Diarrhoea and vomiting
☐ Skin diseases
☐ Undiagnosed lumps and bumps
☐ Localised swelling
☐ Inflammation
☐ Varicose veins
☐ Pregnancy (abdomen)
☐ Cuts
☐ Bruises
☐ Abrasions
☐ Scar tissues (2 years for major operation and 6 months for a small scar)
☐ Sunburn

☐ Hormonal implants
☐ Abdomen (first few days of menstruation depending how the client feels)
☐ Haematoma
☐ Hernia
☐ Recent fractures (minimum 3 months)
☐ Cervical spondylitis
☐ Gastric ulcers
☐ After a heavy meal
☐ Conditions affecting the neck
☐ Any metal pins or plates
☐ Loss of skin sensation (test with tactile test)
☐ IUD (coil)
☐ Anaphylaxis
☐ Muscle fatigue
☐ Pacemaker
☐ Body piercing
☐ Excessive erythema

WRITTEN PERMISSION REQUIRED BY:
☐ GP/Specialist   ☐ Informed consent
Either of which should be attached to the consultation form.

1) **Upper arm**
2) **Waist (across belly button)**
3) **Bust**
4) **Hips (on hip line)**
5) **Thighs**
6) **Calves**

Always ensure you take measurements from the exact same part of the body to prevent error. It is common to mark the client's skin with a non-permanent marker to ensure that re-measurement is taken in the same place .Some spa outlets offer guarantees such as money-back if a certain inch loss is not attained, so accurate measuring is paramount.

PARAFFIN WAX MASK

Paraffin wax is typically applied to the hands and feet for a particularly nourishing and protective manicure or pedicure. It is also used for sports massage treatment to relax and soothe sore and tired muscles.

For this reason a paraffin wax treatment is a particularly luxuriant full body mask, as it combines the moisturising properties of the wax with its muscle-relaxing qualities. Usually a hand or foot cream is applied first so the heat from the paraffin wax increases absorption increasing the overall effects of the treatment.

Special benefits of a paraffin wax mask:

Moisturising

Paraffin wax is particularly effective on dry cracked skin, such as cracked heels or dry elbows, so ensure these areas are generously coated with wax. It can also be combined with other nourishing ingredients which can aid both moisturising qualities and relaxation.

Muscle-relaxing

As paraffin wax is laid onto the skin and hardens slightly. It is renowned for having an ability to aid the healing of injured muscles and reduce swelling and inflammation in joints. This makes it particularly beneficial for clients with conditions such as arthritis, or sports injuries.

Unlike other salon wax which is used for hair removal, paraffin wax is a far softer kind of wax which hardens at a much lower temperature. This means it is fairly soft at room temperature, and can be brushed onto the skin, or used to dip hands and feet. Several layers are often applied to intensify the treatment.

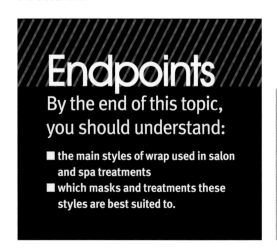

Endpoints
By the end of this topic, you should understand:

■ the main styles of wrap used in salon and spa treatments
■ which masks and treatments these styles are best suited to.

TOPIC 2:
PROFESSIONAL BODY WRAPS

A body wrap is the natural complement to a body mask, and can vary depending on both the underlying mask treatment, and the style of wrap used. Different salons and spas will also have their own methods and favoured ingredients. It is possible, however, to make some general rules as to what constitutes a wrap, and these should always be adhered to when delivering a professional service.

A BODY WRAP CONSISTS OF TWO MAIN ELEMENTS:

1) A mask applied to the skin for the purposes of hydration, detoxification, relaxation, or a combination of these goals.
2) A wrap which acts to increase the efficiency of the mask by adding heat to the treatment, and/or locking in moisture.

Understanding the ingredients/function

Explaining the ingredients and functions of a body wrap is an important part of professional practice. In your place of work you must demonstrate a full understanding of all treatment products and methods of use.

As the spa industry is innovative, treatment product formulations are constantly changing. You should be fully conversant with the specific products used in your spa.

Benefits of wrapping

Therapists use body wraps to enhance the treatment effects of body masks and deliver a number of additional benefits.

- **Increased circulation.** This helps nourish the skin and improve its appearance.
- **Increased perspiration/detoxification.** As explained in detail in Chapter 5: Heat

• KEY POINT

In some cases such as natural wraps, the mask is not a necessary component, but these are the exception rather than the rule.

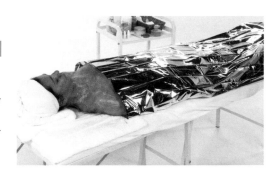

treatments, this draws toxins from the skin and helps speed the flow of lymph.
- **Relaxes tense muscles.** The cocoon-like sensation of being covered in warm wrappings helps the client to relax fully.
- **Temporary weight loss.** In the case of certain bandage wraps, a temporary weight loss can be achieved.
- **Increased absorption.** Therapeutic and emollient ingredients from the underlying mask are absorbed more readily into the skin.

• DID YOU KNOW?

Whilst wraps offer relaxation for clients they should also always offer some additional therapeutic benefit such as detoxification or deep hydration.

Endpoints
By the end of this topic, you should understand:

- the two key components of any body wrap treatment
- the need to understand the ingredients of body wraps you intend to deliver
- benefits of body wrapping as distinct from the benefits of the mask.

TOPIC 3: DIFFERENT WRAP METHODS

Different styles of wrap are teamed with various masks to confer a wide range of benefits for clients. These can range from traditional bandage style body-wraps to those which use plastic or towels. Therapists should bear in mind that specific wrap styles will suit certain masks over others.

The bandage wrap is mainly used for inch-loss. This style of wrap means complete 'mummification' of the body. This is to say that the client is wrapped in bandages from foot to neck and they are wound around the entire body. The bandages themselves are made of stretchy elastic nylon and cotton, allowing them to flex as they are wrapped. This allows very tight application, and leads to particularly effective delivery of treatment.

Depending on the treatment, bandage wraps can go over the top of a mask or themselves be soaked in therapeutic ingredients. In the case of

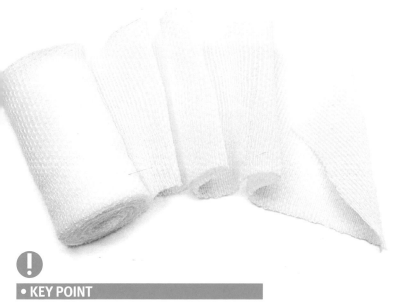

• KEY POINT

A salon or spa would never advertise a wrap based on the method alone. So the term 'bandage-style' wrap would not be known to clients, but rather a 'mud wrap' or 'seaweed wrap', referring to the full treatment of mask and wrap.

• KEY POINT

Although bandage wraps should be applied firmly, they should never be too tight for comfort, or to slow circulation in the skin. Not only would this have the opposite effect of treatment, but more importantly would cause client discomfort.

the mask application underneath, however, the bandages would still be soaked either in additional treatment, or in warm water.

Bandage wraps induce sweating, but their main physical property is to increase circulation and dilation of the capillaries with the firm pressure they direct against the skin.

Wrap-style suited to:
- Detox
- Seaweed.

PLASTIC AND TOWELLING WRAP

This type of wrap is most commonly used in salons and spas. It allows the application of a very wide range of different treatments, from deeply hydrating to detoxifying.

A word about plastic and towelling wrap

Although this style of wrap is not as detoxifying as bandage-style wrapping, it nevertheless induces healthy sweating. In fact the plastic wrapping and loose contact can create more effective sweating than bandages if combined with a heavy blanket.

The plastic and towelling wrap consists of a large thin sheet of plastic which is placed underneath the client on the treatment couch. This plastic can then be arranged around the limbs and body after a mask and exfoliation treatment has taken place. After covering the client in the plastic sheeting towels are folded over the limbs and around the body. It is then usual to add a heavy blanket in order to help further heat the body and so achieve maximum effect.

Wrap-style suited to:
- Essential oils
- Moisturising
- Minerals.

As the name suggests a cocoon wrap sees the client entirely swaddled in towels and blankets in a

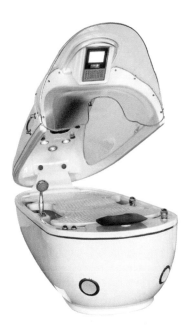

shape resembling a cocoon or chrysalis.

Oversized blankets and towels are placed beneath the client prior to treatment application. The towels and blankets are then folded carefully around the body in a number of layers to maximise the warmth and relaxation of the client. The end result is for all the blankets to be tucked neatly into place, alongside an extra towel which encompasses the head and forehead. The face is uncovered.

Wrap-style suited to:
- Herbal wrap
- Medical wraps (such as hot and cool wraps)
- Moisturising/relaxing.

Endpoints
By the end of this topic, you should understand:

- the main styles of wrap used in salon and spa treatments
- which masks and treatments these styles are best suited to.

TOPIC 4: NATURAL WRAPS

Many wrap treatments are applied with a mask, but it is also possible to apply a 'natural' wrap which uses only thermal (hot/cold) properties to treat. They rely on the properties of the wrapping material to heat or cool the body, and knowledge of which area of the body the wrap should be applied to.

DRY BLANKET WRAP
This wrap is designed for the simple purpose of inducing healthy perspiration. It is particularly beneficial for weaker clients (such as the elderly), and those suffering chronic joint-pain conditions such as arthritis. It is also useful for clients with sensitive skin.

Equipment needed includes:
- Linen sheets
- A thick wool or thermal blanket
- Hot water bottles
- Large towels
- A small towel to act as a cold compress.

1) Prior to treatment the client takes a hot body bath or hot foot bath for fifteen to thirty minutes with a cold compress applied to the forehead.
2) During treatment, the client is wrapped entirely in warm towels and blankets, with hot water bottles applied to feet and at the sides. A cold compress is applied to the forehead.
3) The client rests in the wrap for thirty minutes. Treatment can be optionally followed by a full cold bath or shower for thirty seconds to a minute.

A word about natural wraps

Natural wraps are more commonly found in medical-style spas than in day-spas or location-spas. Whilst they can be very relaxing applied as a solo treatment, established practice is to use them as part of a much longer treatment involving several stages such as massage and hydrotherapy.

COOL MOIST BLANKET BODY WRAP

A cooling wrap which can be used to reduce and draw out excess body heat, and can be teamed with a perspiration-inducing hot tea such as peppermint. It is beneficial for those with nervous dispositions, skin ailments and elevated body temperature.

It is also useful for introducing hot and cold temperature variation with clients for whom a Swiss bath or shower is otherwise unsuitable.

1) The wrap consists of a long double body compress with a layer of cloth separating the legs. These are prepared in cold (but not iced) water and wrung out so as to be damp rather than soaking wet.

2) Prior to the wrap the client takes either a hot bath or a hot foot bath. As they emerge the cold sheet is placed over the couch so as to maximise the retention of the cold temperature.

3) The client is then rapidly wrapped in the sheet and a cold compress left on the forehead. Treatment lasts between fifteen and thirty minutes. The body can be optionally rubbed with diluted vinegar at the end of treatment to aid detoxification.

MEDICAL WRAPS

Some wraps are designed for medical as well as relaxation or beauty purposes. It is unlikely you will encounter these styles of wrap in the UK, but therapists practising in areas such as Switzerland and Eastern Europe may encounter modifications of wraps to directly treat certain areas.

Areas of the body where wraps can be used include:

1) **Calves and feet.** These are the most common type of wrap which are used on only one area of the body. As the calves and feet have lower circulation a hot or cold wrap to this area can stimulate blood flow and promote health. Techniques include bandage-style wraps or specialist knee-socks which can be soaked before application.

2) **Chest wrap.** For breathing disorders such as bronchitis, inflammation, or damage caused by smoking a chest wrap can be employed. Cotton and linen cloths are wrapped right around the chest and a cold compress applied to the head.

3) **Throat wrap.** Throat inflammation can be treated this way, usually by a cold wrap. Thick linen cloths are wound around the throat area after pre-soaking in cold water.

A word about medical wraps

Whilst hot and cold wraps can be used on certain parts of the body, any serious ailment should be referred to a GP. Never try to treat a condition which is causing a client significant pain or discomfort and has not been subject to professional medical examination. Refer to the list of contraindications if you are unsure.

Endpoints

By the end of this topic, you should understand:

- the possibility of using a 'natural' wrap without a mask treatment
- applications of natural wraps
- use of varying temperatures to enact key benefits of natural wraps
- likely applications and treatment environs of natural wrap treatments.

TOPIC 5:
APPLYING A STANDARD PROFESSIONAL WRAP

At its core a body wrap is simple in nature and although there are a variety of different wraps available to clients, they can be found in many spas.

Whilst the treatment can be straight-forward, however, your skill as a therapist will ensure that this spa treatment will be a memorable and effective one for the client. It is your professionalism, as well as the seamless manner in which you guide the client through the various stages of the wrap, that will make the difference to the client's overall spa experience.

APPLYING A STANDARD PLASTIC WRAP WITH MASK

Checklist: Equipment for wrap application
- Spa treatment set-up with be, towels and linens
- Plastic sheeting
- Extra towels or sponges to remove product if no shower is present
- Body mask (seaweed, mud, etc.)
- Cleanser and toner if used (face only)
- Moisturiser to suit mask
- Water
- Thermal blanket
- Large brush to paint on product OR gloves for hand application.

Wraps involve many different stages, many of which involve skill in combining with a relaxing ambiance.

This mask uses standard plastic and blanket wrapping. Masks which use bandages vary slightly in their application, although the preparatory steps and after care are the same.

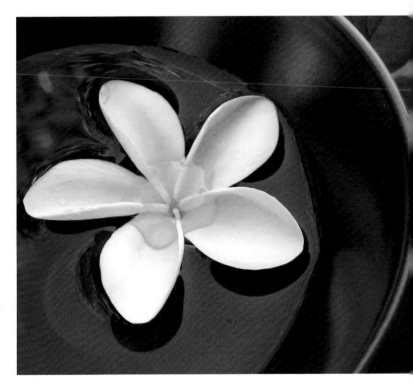

PREPARATION
1) **Preparing the room**. Before the client even enters the room it should be correctly equipped with the towels and protective elements necessary. As you will be applying a full mask the entire couch must be covered with plastic protective sheeting, and possibly parts of the flooring.
2) **Preparing the couch**. Well before the client enters the room the couch should be pre-covered with the material in which you will wrap them. On top of this you should place a heavy sheet. The client will lie on top of the wrap and under the top-sheet as you apply their mask, ready to be wrapped without leaving the couch.

3) **Preparing the shower area**. If you have a treatment room with a shower inside, ensure this is clean with adequate robes and towels. If the client needs to enter an adjoining room, you will need to check that their route will not disturb other treatments, or that they themselves will not be encountering other clients.

4) **Adding any necessary equipment**. Have the mask you will be using and any other products used to remove the mask or deliver massage during the treatment. Ensure disposable underwear and a plastic shower-cap is in the room for the client to wear during the wrap. Warm the mask if this is directed by the manufacturer.

5) **Attending to the ambiance**. Many therapists like to prepare the working environment with the use of colour, essential oils or candles and soothing music. How you decide on this will be down to either your preference, or the spa philosophy. You should always remember, however, that it is often the small extra touches which add real professionalism to your service.

6) **Consult the client** to ascertain suitability and reasons for treatment paying particular attention to any contraindications (see consultation form).

7) **Wash your hands**.

CONSULTATION AND CONTRAINDICATIONS

Any medical complaint should be referred to a GP if you are unsure. Below is a list of contraindications which would render a client unsuited to a wrap treatment.

In circumstances where written medical permission cannot be obtained the client must sign an informed consent form stating that the treatment and its effects have been fully explained to them and confirm that they are willing to proceed without permission from their GP or specialist.

- **Pregnancy**
- **Cardio vascular conditions (thrombosis, phlebitis, hypertension, hypotension, heart conditions)**
- **Haemophilia**
- **Medical oedema**
- **Osteoporosis**

- **Arthritis**
- **Nervous/psychotic conditions**
- **Epilepsy**
- **Recent operations**
- **Diabetes**
- **Asthma**
- **Any dysfunction of the nervous system (e.g. muscular sclerosis, Parkinson's disease, motor neurone disease)**
- **Trapped/pinched nerve (e.g. sciatica)**
- **Inflamed nerve**
- **Cancer**
- **Postural deformities**
- **Spastic conditions**
- **Kidney infections**
- **Whiplash**
- **Slipped disc**
- **Undiagnosed pain**
- **When taking prescribed medication**
- **Acute rheumatism**
- **Any condition already being treated by a GP or another complementary practitioner**
- **Fever**
- **Contagious or infectious diseases**
- **Under the influence of recreational drugs or alcohol**
- **Diarrhoea and vomiting**
- **Skin diseases**
- **Undiagnosed lumps and bumps**
- **Localised swelling**
- **Inflammation**
- **Varicose veins**
- **Pregnancy (abdomen)**
- **Cuts**
- **Bruises**
- **Abrasions**
- **Scar tissues (two years for major operation and six months for a small scar)**
- **Sunburn**
- **Hormonal implants**
- **Abdomen (first few days of menstruation depending how the client feels)**
- **Haematoma**
- **Hernia**
- **Recent fractures (minimum three months)**
- **Cervical spondylitis**
- **Gastric ulcers**
- **After a heavy meal**
- **Conditions affecting the neck.**

EXPLAINING TREATMENT TO THE CLIENT

1) Talk the client through what will happen at every stage of the process. Double-check they are happy with the procedure and offer to answer any questions they may have.

2) Make a special point of mentioning the attention you intend to pay to the client's modesty. They will be in underwear – most likely disposable underwear provided by the spa. A thorough explanation of the treatment and procedures should prevent any unnecessary embarrassment on behalf of the client with respect to body exposure. It is important to reassure them throughout the treatment and keep them informed throughout the whole process.

3) Ask the client if they would like the mask applied to the chest and stomach area. If you are applying a wrap for weight-loss, the chest will often yield good inch-loss, so this point can be made to the client if necessary.

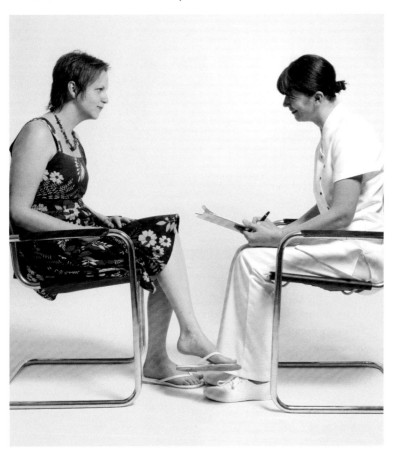

GUIDING THE CLIENT THROUGH TREATMENT:

Stage one: Preparing the body

1) Allow the client to enter the room first and explain that they may remove their clothes here. Point out to them disposable underwear for their use, and a robe for them to wear whilst they await your return.

2) Explain there is also a plastic shower-cap to protect their hair during treatment.

3) Explain that they should lie on their back on the couch under the top sheet.

4) Leave the room and time five minutes before your return.

5) Re-enter and adjust any areas of top-sheet which are not straight. Also check the shower-cap is comfortably fitted and adequately covering the client's hair as it can often slip as they move themselves under the top-sheet.

6) Cleanse the feet using a medi-wipe or similar.

7) Optional. Cleanse and tone the skin.

8) Perform a pre-treatment exfoliation (see Chapter 3: Exfoliation). This is most likely to be a body-brush or loofah exfoliation rather than a scrub, but will depend on the wrap being applied.

Stage 2: Applying the mask and wrap

1) Have the client cross their arms to hold the top-sheet in place and sit up on the couch, exposing their back.

2) Take the warmed mask and apply generously to the entire back, using either your hands or a large brush. Gloves can be worn.

3) Guide the client to lie back on the couch and apply the mask to the shoulder and upper chest area.

4) Apply the mask to the arms one at a time from shoulder to hand.

5) If the client has indicated they are comfortable with having the mask applied to their chest and stomach gently lower the top sheet, and layer the mask around the breasts and over the stomach in a circular motion.

6 Cover the upper part of the body.

7) Raise the nearest leg to where you are standing and apply the mask to the underside and up over the buttocks. Ease the leg back down and sweep the mask over the front of the leg. Wrap

the leg in the plastic sheeting.

8) Move around the couch and repeat the process on the other leg.

9) Some types of wrap/mask are applied with the client prone initially. The mask is applied to the whole of the back of the body first. The client is then asked to turn over and the mask is applied to the entire front of the body, excluding the face. The plastic sheeting and additional coverings may then be folded according to manufacturer's instructions.

Stage 3: Wrapping the client and removing treatment

1) The client is now encased in the first layer of plastic wrap and should now be entirely swaddled in blankets or towels to enable warmth and relaxation for optimal treatment.

2) If using towels, move the towels from under the client to lay them over the top. Pull them quite tight against the body for a cocoon effect. If necessary add extra towels to the top.

3) If using a blanket cover the client entirely with a heavy blanket. Thermal blankets can also be used.

4) Verbally check that the client is comfortable.

5) If the client is on a heated bed, this is the stage at which to turn on the power supply and allow the warmth to rise up from under the client.

6) Either: stay with the client throughout the treatment (usually twenty-five minutes) remaining quiet as they relax.

7) Or: if specified as part of the treatment, deliver an additional treatment whilst the mask is taking effect, such as face and scalp massage.

Stage 4a: Removing the product – with shower facility

1) If your facility has a shower, begin to fold away the towels or remove the blanket, starting with the legs, but keep the central towel in place for modesty.

2) Fold away the plastic sheeting, leaving the central towel in place.

3) Direct the client to enter the shower when you leave the room, keeping their shower-cap in place. Explain the location of robes for them to use after their shower.

4) If applying lotion following the treatment direct

● KEY POINT

Regularly check in with your client with regards to temperature and comfort.

the client to lie back on the couch following their shower. If no lotion is to be applied the client can dress and the treatment concluded.

5) Exit the room for ten minutes.

6) Re-enter and either apply lotion area by area, or conclude the treatment.

Stage 4b: Removing the product – without shower facility

Many smaller outlets do not have en-suite shower facilities as part of their treatment rooms. This is by no means a barrier to professional treatment and many clients prefer having their mask removed manually by the therapist. You must ensure, however, that all parts of the mask are adequately removed, particularly around areas such as the chest and head which will be on public display when the client exits the salon.

1) As part of your preparation of the room, ensure adequate towels and warm water are available.

2) In the reverse order to which you applied the mask, carefully wipe away the mask from the skin using damp warm towels.

3) Continue until all the mask is removed and double check for areas such as behind the knee, ears and in the crease of the arm where treatment can be harder to wipe away.

4) Progress to the next stage of the treatment such as moisturising as applicable.

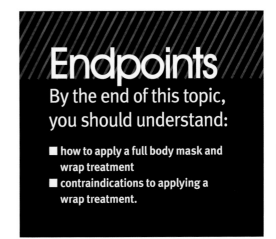

Endpoints
By the end of this topic, you should understand:

■ **how to apply a full body mask and wrap treatment**

■ **contraindications to applying a wrap treatment.**

TOPIC 6:
ADAPTATING WRAPS TO YOUR CLIENT

Wraps are intensive treatments and can come with a variety of contraindications. As they are a heat treatment in many ways, contraindications for this area will apply, alongside the usual spectrum of allergies and skin conditions which you would usually run through with a client receiving a facial treatment.

TAILORING THE TREATMENT TO THE CLIENT

Part of the therapist's skill will be adapting and matching the wide range of wrap treatments to the differing needs of clients. Generally, however, wraps fall into three broad categories of those seeking treatment.

Relaxation

This client is seeking mostly the relaxing and restorative properties of the wrap. They should be encouraged to try moisturising-style wraps and skin enriching wraps rather than stimulating or detoxifying treatments. Similarly, they suit treatments which include relaxing massage such as scalp or facial massage.

Moisturising

This client may be teamed with either a moisturising wrap or a seaweed/mud wrap often to good effect. Both offer skin nourishing and enriching qualities, but you will need to question the client as to which effects they would rather gain – relaxation or detoxification – to accompany the moisturising effect.

Detoxification

This client is seeking detoxification, but more usually actual inch and weight loss as the result of their wrap. If you do not offer the bandage-style seaweed and mud wraps but instead use a more general detoxification treatment it is important to explain to the client that this wrap has health benefits but inch-loss will not be measured. Similarly a moisturising wrap would not be appropriate as they would not confer the expected result to the client.

Endpoints

By the end of this topic, you should understand:

- how to match a client to a wrap and/or mask treatment
- the three main categories of client for mask and wrap treatment.

09

Massage techniques

Massage is the manipulation of the soft tissues of the body, leading to benefits for all the body systems. The techniques in this book, which are based on the Swedish system, use the application of pressure to either soothe or stimulate.

TOPIC 1: MASSAGE TECHNIQUES

WHAT IS MASSAGE?

Massage is a combination of various movements used to manipulate tissues for both local and overall effects and benefits. The movements range from gentle stroking to invigorating friction, depending on the desired effect. Massage is generally based on the Swedish system and several types of massage have developed which incorporate these techniques for different therapeutic effects.

What is Swedish massage?

The Swedish system of massage is named after the man who developed it, Per Henrik Ling. He was a physiologist and fencing master and developed a system of movements which he found helpful for improving his health and maintaining his physical condition. Classical massage is still based on the techniques he used, i.e. effleurage, petrissage and percussion. This chapter will look at these fundamental movements as well as variations of them.

EFFLEURAGE
What is effleurage?

The name effleurage derives from *effleurer*, a French word meaning 'to touch lightly'. It is generally a gentle, sweeping, relaxing stroke, with varying levels of pressure, used at the beginning and end of a massage. It can also be used with firm pressure over large areas once the muscles are relaxed. Unlike petrissage and percussion, effleurage does not aim to move or manipulate tissues or muscles, only to soothe and relax them and improve circulation.

How to do it

With fingers and thumbs together, keep the hands relaxed and stroke the skin slowly and rhythmically with a confident pressure. When massaging the

limbs, the emphasis of the pressure is towards the heart. The hands may be used one after the other or at the same time. The whole palm of the hand and the fingers should be used to prevent tickling the client. Hands must mould to the contours of the area being treated. Once a gentle rhythm has been established the therapist can increase the pressure gradually to prepare the body for the deeper work that follows.

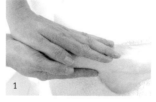
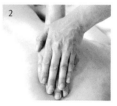
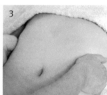
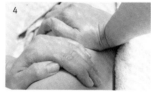
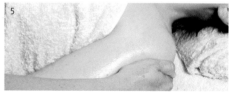

When to use it

Effleurage is used at the start and finish of a massage session and at the start and finish of each body part, e.g. at the beginning and end of work on the back or legs. It is also used as a connection stroke between different parts of the massage. When carrying out a massage the therapist must not break contact with the client because when the hands are removed the client's body senses this, believes the massage is over and begins to rouse itself from its relaxed state.

What does it do?

As the first contact between therapist and client, effleurage helps to prepare the body for massage, introducing the client to the therapist's touch, spreading the massage medium such as oil or cream (if used), warming the skin and relaxing the client. It is also used after more invigorating strokes to help the elimination of toxins from the areas that have been worked. It can also help desquamation, especially when used deeply, and thus help the skin to regenerate.

Effleurage on the limbs with the pressure working towards the heart assists the return of blood to the heart and aids lymph drainage. Deep effleurage also pushes blood into superficial capillaries.

What are the contraindications to massage?

Massage is non-invasive, relaxing and natural. It is therefore generally considered a safe treatment for most people. However, there are two types of contraindication: with GP, medical or specialist permission and contraindications that restrict treatment.

With medical, GP or specialist permission – in circumstances where written medical permission cannot be obtained the client must sign an informed consent stating that the treatment and its effect has been fully explained to them and confirm that they are willing to proceed without permission from their GP or specialist.

- Pregnancy
- Cardio vascular conditions (thrombosis, phlebitis, hypertension, hypotension, heart conditions)
- Haemophilia
- Any condition already being treated by a GP or another complementary practitioner
- Medical oedema
- Osteoporosis
- Arthritis
- Nervous/psychotic conditions
- Epilepsy
- Recent operations
- Diabetes
- Asthma
- Any dysfunction of the nervous system (e.g. muscular sclerosis, Parkinson's disease, motor neurone disease)
- Bell's palsy
- Trapped/pinched nerve (e.g. sciatica)
- Inflamed nerve

● REMEMBER

Effleurage is a relaxing stroke that is used to prepare the body for deeper techniques.

- Cancer
- Postural deformities
- Cervical spondylitis
- Spastic conditions
- Kidney infections
- Whiplash
- Slipped disc
- Undiagnosed pain
- When taking prescribed medication
- Acute rheumatism

Contraindications that restrict treatment
- Fever
- Contagious or infectious diseases
- Under the influence of recreational drugs or alcohol
- Diarrhoea and vomiting
- Skin diseases
- Undiagnosed lumps and bumps
- Localised swelling
- Inflammation
- Varicose veins
- Pregnancy (abdomen)
- Cuts
- Bruises
- Abrasions
- Scar tissues (two years for major operation and six months for a small scar)
- Sunburn
- Hormonal implants
- Menstruation (abdomen – first few days)
- Haematoma
- Hernia
- Recent fractures (minimum three months)
- Gastric ulcers
- After a heavy meal
- Conditions affecting the neck

Does a contraindication mean that treatment cannot take place?

Not always. However, in the above cases and whenever you are unsure whether it is safe to proceed, it is best to refer the client to their GP for advice. The therapist should not, under any circumstances, attempt to diagnose a condition or decide whether an existing condition is treatable. The code of conduct of many complementary health associations states that diagnosis is not allowed. If there is any uncertainty, refer the client.

PETRISSAGE
What is petrissage?

Petrissage, like effleurage, is a name derived from French. *Pétrir* means to knead or rub with force and this stroke uses both kneading and rubbing movements to manipulate tissues and muscles. It uses the pressure of the hands or fingers to break down tension. There are various methods: in some cases only the fingers and/or thumbs are used to knead the tissues, in others the whole hand is used.

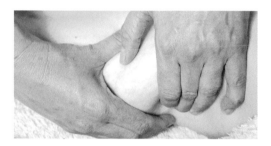

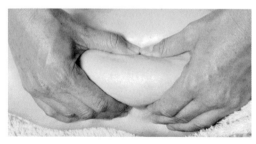

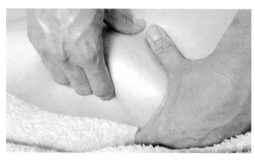

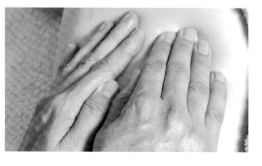

KNEADING

Carefully and slowly grasp the flesh of the part of the body being worked with both hands or fingers then use one hand to lift it, as if pulling it away from the bone. Keep the tissues firmly compressed whilst lifting, then release and repeat with the other hand. Continue to lift, compress and release with alternate hands, as if kneading dough and build up into a rhythm. For particularly stiff/tight areas, build a twist into the movement so that the flesh is being 'wrung' like a damp cloth. The pressure should be smooth and not jerky and care should be taken to avoid pinching the skin. Begin gently and build up to firmer pressure, always using the same rate and rhythm and getting feedback from the client. It is important to use body weight and movement to assist in making the technique effective and less tiring for the therapist. Lean into the muscle as you grasp it and lean back as you lift.

When to use it

Petrissage usually follows effleurage at the start of a massage. It should be used to break down tightness and tension in large muscles. It should not be used on bony or delicate areas.

What does it do?

Kneading stretches the muscles, and compresses tissue against tissue improving suppleness and elasticity, and helps break down tension and stiffness in tissues and large muscles. Such stiffness is often caused by the build-up of toxins such as lactic acid. Kneading helps to release and break down these toxins, enabling the muscles to work more efficiently.

● REMEMBER

Petrissage (or kneading) is a firm application of pressure which compresses tissue against tissue, thus releasing muscle tightness and breaking down toxins and tension. It also stimulates the circulation. Despite the firmness of the stroke it is more relaxing than invigorating because it releases any tight muscles and the toxins within.

FRICTION

The name friction, like many others used in massage, comes from a Latin word, *fricare*, which means to rub or rub down. Friction techniques are all variations of rubbing and they work by compressing tissue against bone. It is often used for close work on a small area or on specific areas of tightness.

How to do it

Place thumbs or fingers, particularly the balls/pads of the thumb, on the section of the body to be worked on. Apply firm pressure from your body and circle the tissue immediately below the thumbs slowly and deeply. Try to imagine the tissues below the surface of the skin and how the rubbing movement pushes them against other muscles and against the bones creating friction. The thumbs can be rubbed up and down or held in a static position. Fingertips can also be used if the therapist finds them more effective. Once the small area has been thoroughly worked move to another section. The therapist should not be moving rapidly across an expanse of flesh but deliberately and slowly focusing on a small section at a time, moving along the length of a muscle. Depending on the type of skin/individual's requirements the therapist will need to adjust the length of time spent on each small area in order to prevent rubbing for too long and causing soreness. The effect should be one of heat and tension.

Cross-fibre friction is a variation of this technique in which the therapist works across the muscle at right angles to the fibres instead of along the length of the muscle. This helps to stretch the muscle fibres and release tension. It is used extensively by physiotherapists and sports massage therapists in the treatment of injuries.

When to use it

Friction is a method used for focusing on a particular problem area. It is especially useful for releasing tension in muscles and for loosening tightness around joints. It is not recommended for use all over the body because it is time-consuming and tiring for the therapist. It is also used on small muscles where petrissage is not appropriate. On tight muscles friction can be very painful, so caution is vital in the care of the client.

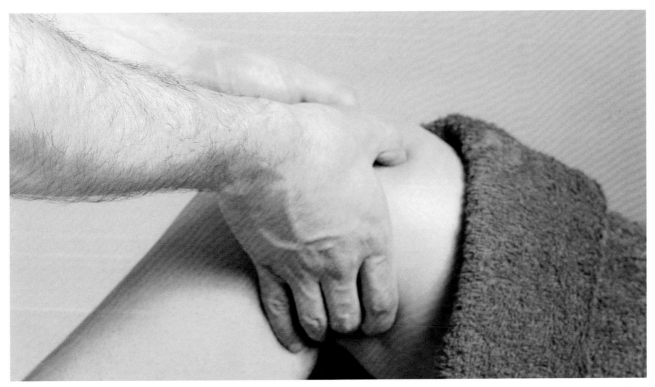

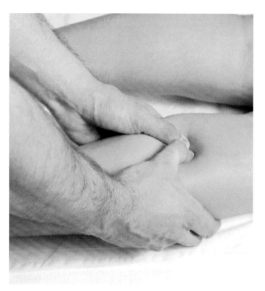

● REMEMBER

Frictions are firm rubbing and heat-producing techniques which compress tissue against bone. They are used for close work on areas of tension or by physiotherapists or sports massage therapists in treating injury.

FRICTION
What does it do?

Friction movements heat up the local area, improve circulation, promote lymph drainage, stimulate the nerves and loosen tightness in the muscles. Working very closely with the muscles helps to break down any local 'knottiness' or lumpiness. Cross-fibre friction helps stretch the muscle fibres and release any tension held in the muscle; it also allows the therapist, particularly in sports massage, to work close to a damaged or inflamed area without touching it, because working on one section of muscle helps stretch the rest of the muscle.

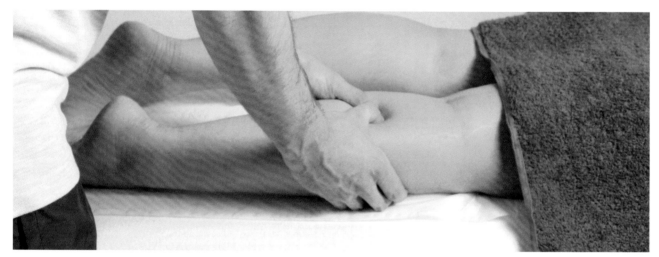

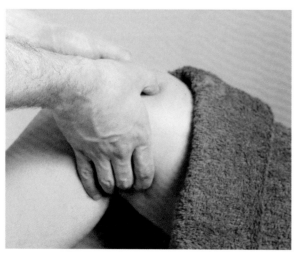

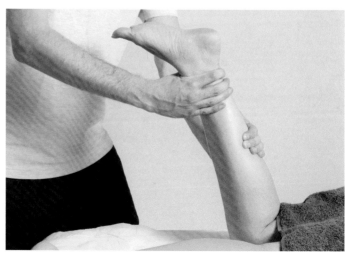

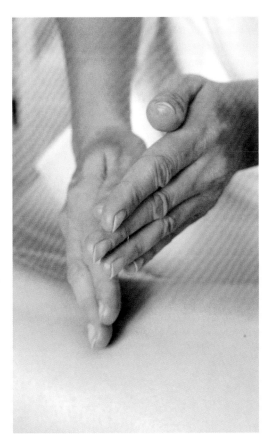

PERCUSSION
What is percussion?

Percussion derives from the Latin word *percutere* meaning to hit. Percussion techniques are brisk, invigorating and stimulating strokes, which use the hands to strike the body rapidly and suddenly. The classic 'chopping' motion associated with Swedish massage is a percussion technique called hacking. The others are pounding, beating, cupping and tapotement.

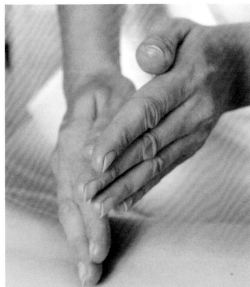

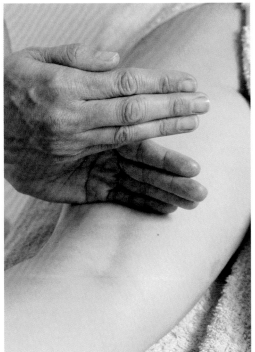

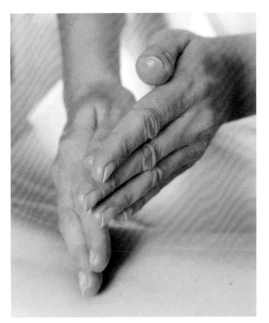

A classic massage technique called hacking

DID YOU KNOW?

Percutere (the origin of the word percussion) can be broken down into per meaning through and *quatere* means to shake. Percussion thus means a shaking through the body.

How to do it

Hacking: hold both hands over the body with palms facing each other and the edge of the little finger closest to the client. The fingers should be together and relaxed and the elbows out, away from the body. Strike the body with alternate hands, with the movement originating from the wrist. As soon as one hand touches the skin let it spring back as the other drops to hack. Begin slowly with a light pressure and build up to a vigorous rhythm with firm pressure. Keep the hands and wrists relaxed to prevent causing pain and keep the rhythm bouncy and light.

● REMEMBER

Percussion is a striking, wake-up stroke. It has a stimulating action on the tissues.

Beating: make hands into fists, with the little finger side facing each other. Lower one fist then the other alternately, lifting one fist as the other lowers. Begin slowly with a light pressure and build up to a vigorous rhythm with firm pressure. Keep both hands and wrists relaxed and keep the movement brisk and springy so that the fists bounce away from the body as soon as they touch it and do not thump or cause pain. Pounding should only be used on fleshy areas.

Pounding: similar to beating except the sides of the fist hit the tissue and the little finger side of the fist faces down towards the clients skin.

Cupping: hold hands out with palm facing up then form 'cup' shapes with the hands. Invert the 'cups' so that the 'inside' is closest to the client's skin. Then, following the same rhythm as hacking, lower one 'cup' then the next alternately. Begin slowly with light pressure and build up to a vigorous rhythm with firm pressure. Keep both hands and wrists relaxed and keep the movement brisk and springy. If done properly, the movement will create a sound similar to the 'clip clop' of horses hooves. As air is pushed away from the surface of the skin by the pressure of the cupped hands, thus creating a vacuum.

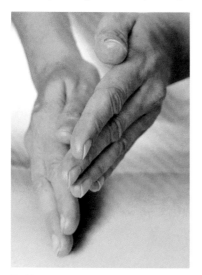

Hacking

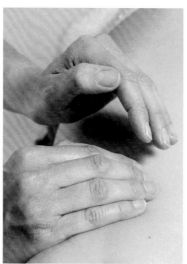

Cupping:

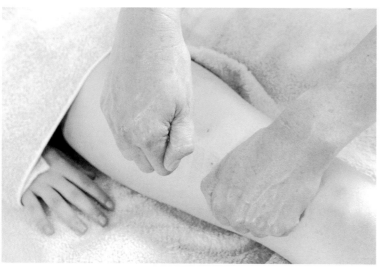

Beating

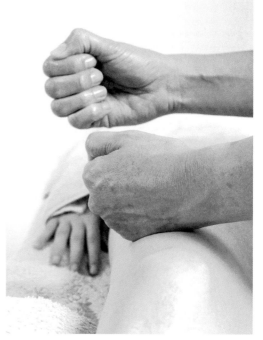

Pounding

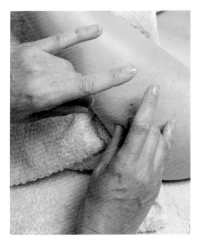
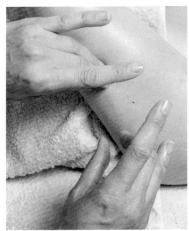

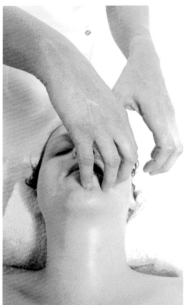
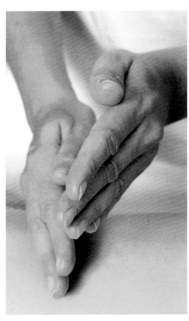

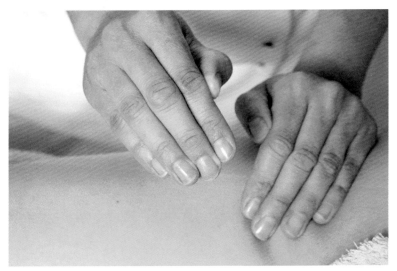

Be careful not to slap.

It is the coming off the body with suction that stimulates the systems of the body, particularly the cardiovascular system. A redness, or erythema, may develop.

Tapotement: this is a very gentle form of percussion, using just the fingertips, which is carried out on delicate or sensitive areas, such as the face. The name derives from tapoter, a French word meaning to tap, and tapping is the basis of the technique. Keep the fingers loose and relaxed and tap the area very lightly and gently. Start slowly and build up to a gentle, repetitive and firm rhythm. As with other percussion movements the hands should be relaxed in order to keep the stroke bouncy. This is a soothing movement and should not be heavy or jerky.

When to use it

Percussion should be used as an invigorating, wake-up stroke. If the aim of the whole massage is to stimulate the system rather than soothe it, percussion should form the major part of the treatment. If the aim of the massage is to soothe or relax, percussion can be used towards the end of the treatment, before the final effleurage strokes, to 'wake up' the client's systems. It should not be used on bony or delicate areas.

What does it do?

Percussion is the most invigorating of massage techniques. It improves local and overall circulation, warms the skin and muscles, improves muscle tone both because of the physical effect of the treatment and because of the improved circulation, helps break up fat deposits in fleshy areas and invigorates the nerves.

● REMEMBER

Percussion is a striking, wake-up stroke. It has a stimulating action on the tissues.

OTHER TECHNIQUES
What is vibration?

Vibration can be either manual or mechanical. It aims to make the muscle tremble and shake in order to loosen tightness and release tension. Mechanical vibration equipment can be used to produce the same effects.

How to do it

Vibration can be carried out using either one or both hands and either whole palms or just the fingertips. Place the palms of the hands/fingertips on the muscle and, retaining firm, deep contact with the muscle throughout the movement, briskly move the hands/fingertips up and down or from side to side by tensing the arms so much that they shake.

When to use it

When muscles are extremely tight and not responding well to petrissage or frictions.

What does it do?

Vibration helps release pain and tension. It can be a very soothing technique or a very stimulating one, depending on the desired result. It can literally surprise the muscle into releasing its tension.

Passive joint movements

Passive movements require the client to relax and let the therapist gently take a joint (e.g. knee, elbow, shoulder) through its natural range of movement. These movements may help to improve mobility and release tension.

● REMEMBER

Vibration is a pain reliever which clears nerve pathways and helps loosen tightness in the muscles.

● REMEMBER

- Massage movements should always be used with upward pressure towards the heart. This helps venous return and lymphatic drainage.
- During a massage session the therapist should always aim to keep at least one hand in contact with the client, to prevent interrupting the mood of relaxation, and to reassure the client.
- Percussion and petrissage should not be used on bony or delicate areas.
- The therapist should start with light strokes and gentle pressure and build up to deeper strokes and firmer pressure, whilst maintaining a slow rate and rhythm throughout.

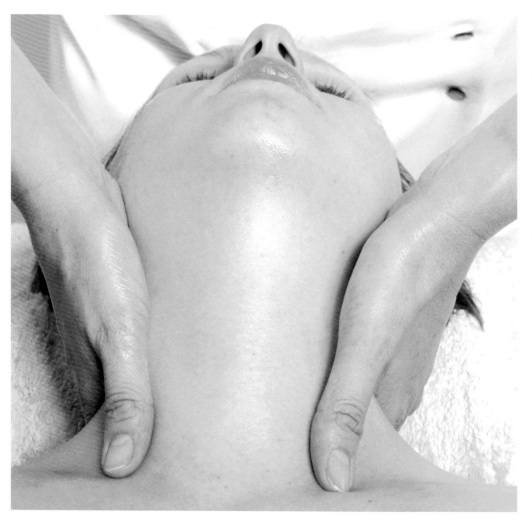

GENERAL SUMMARY
Massage techniques and effects

The following is a general summary of the styles of movement or pressure used in massage and their effects on the body. It is intended as a guideline, not an absolute. With some treatments and some clients different effects may result and the techniques may be used differently.

How do I use the techniques in a routine?
The therapist's routine

Per Ling used the following routine: effleurage, petrissage, effleurage, percussion, effleurage. However, all massage therapists will develop their own routines according to the requirements of their clients. The therapist is the source of the massage and thus can control its effects and results. It is the therapist's responsibility to find out about the client's requirements and expectations and plan a routine that will meet them. For example, a client who wants a thorough, invigorating massage will require a routine built around stimulating techniques such as percussion with less focus on relaxing, gentle strokes like effleurage. A client who wants a relaxing massage will require a routine that focuses on effleurage and petrissage with less emphasis on percussion, if it is used at all. Mechanical methods are generally not used in relaxation because they are not as effective as the hands, either for palpating the muscles or for relaxing the client through touch. The time spent on each type of movement and the pressure used will also be determined by the individual's needs and the desired results.

The client's input

Each individual will experience massage techniques differently so that one may find a percussion movement very invigorating whereas another finds it painful. Again the therapist must work with the client to achieve the best results. The aim is to invigorate and/or soothe and at no time should the client's comments, especially with respect to pain, be ignored. The therapist must learn to adapt to each client's pain threshold. Ignoring it will in the short-term prevent the massage from being relaxing and in the long-term may cause damage.

Why are continuous movements necessary?

One hand or both should always be kept on the body during treatment since as soon as the hands are removed the body will register this as the end of the massage and begin to 'change gear', getting ready to dress and leave.

Endpoints
By the end of this topic, you should understand:

- the classic Swedish massage techniques, how to use them and why. The next section explains other massage techniques
- the different techniques used in massage, how and when to perform them and what they do
- the importance of the therapist's input and that of the client. The next section explains what a massage medium is and why it is used.

TOPIC 2: MASSAGE MEDIUMS

What is a massage medium?

A massage medium is a lubricant which helps the therapist's hands to move freely and smoothly over the client's skin. The three most common mediums used are oil, cream and powder.

Massage oils

Oil is the most useful massage medium because it is smooth and light. Massage oils should be of vegetable or plant origin and not too thick or heavy because the heat and pressure of massage movements can make them sticky. Lighter oils, such as grapeseed, are more useful for larger areas because they are smoother. Thicker oils, such as avocado are more useful for smaller areas. Blends of oils can be used either for a blend of properties or to make a more expensive oil go further, e.g. a dense, expensive oil such as evening primrose oil, which is very good for use on dry skin, could be blended with a lighter, less expensive oil such as grapeseed. Mineral oils, such as baby oil, should not be used as they dry the skin.

Massage creams

Creams are good for small or delicate areas such as the face or on very dry skin. They tend to be heavier and more oily than oils. As they are absorbed faster than massage oils, they may require more frequent application.

Powder

Powder is useful for oily skin, very hairy clients or on clients who dislike the residues of oils and creams. Swedish massage was traditionally performed using powder because powder prevents the hands from sliding over the surface of the body and allows deeper pressure.

How much medium should I use?

The amount of medium used will depend on the client. In general a full body massage will require about 20-25ml of oil. Massage of larger clients and those with dry skin will require more medium.

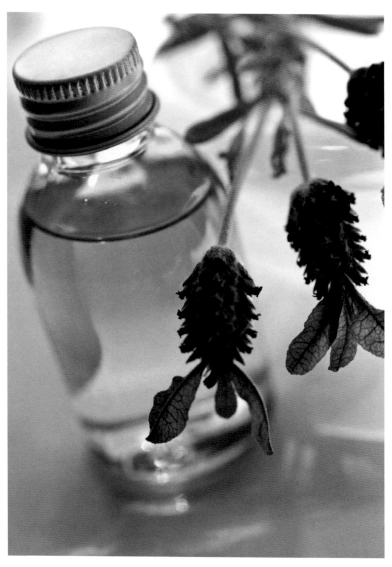

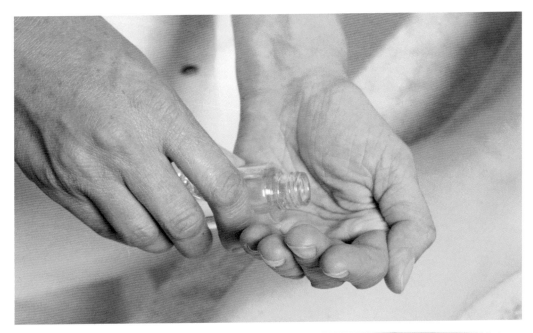

How do I apply it?

All massage mediums should first be dispensed into the therapist's hands, rather than straight on to the client's body. This is because the oil, cream or powder will be cold and uncomfortable on the skin if it is not warmed up and evenly distributed. The therapist should dispense a small amount into the palm of one hand and then rub the hands together to warm the medium and distribute it smoothly across palms and fingertips. The therapist should then apply the medium using effleurage strokes.

Sensitive skin and allergies

Before using any oil, cream or powder, the therapist may wish to carry out a patch test, especially if the client has sensitive skin or allergies. Wash the crook of the elbow with water or water and a mild soap, dry it then rub a small amount of the medium onto the skin. Leave for 24 hours and check for any reactions.

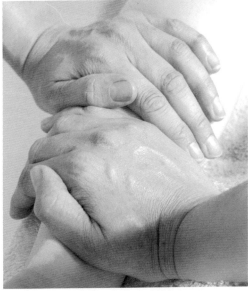

One possible method for applying oil

Endpoints

By the end of this topic, you should understand:

■ the different techniques and mediums used in massage.

Topic 3: Massage routine

Please also see the fully interactive CDROM for the full routine

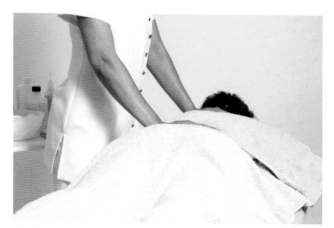

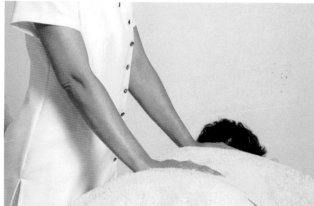

Holding on the back

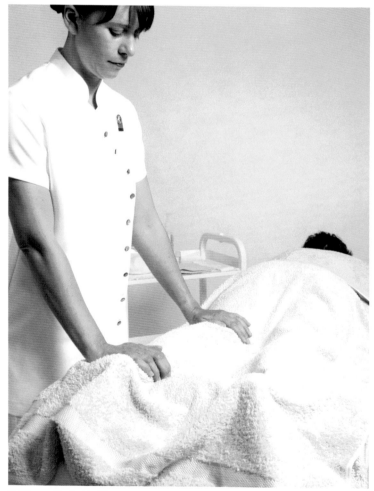

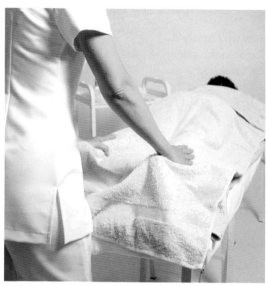

Slowly turn back the towels

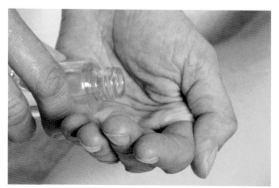

Holding on the feet/ankles

Pouring the oil

BACK OF THE LEGS

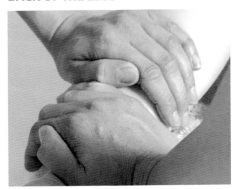 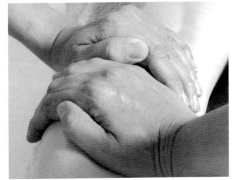

1) Effleurage to spread the oil

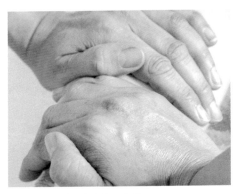 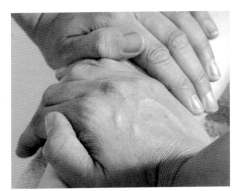

2) Effleurage the whole leg six times

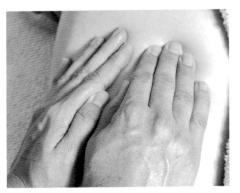 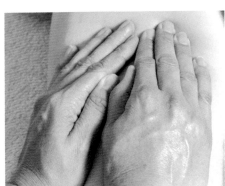

3) Palmar kneading to the back of the thigh six times

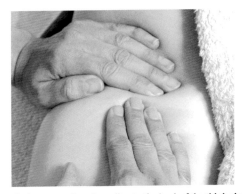 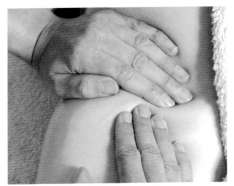

4) Alternate palmar kneading to the back of the thigh six times

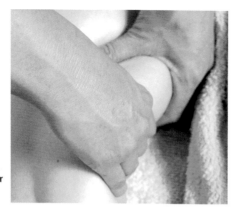
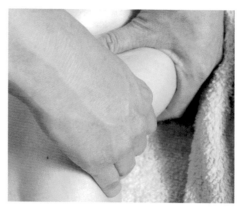

5) Picking up twice all over the back of the thigh

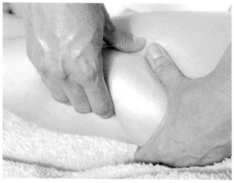
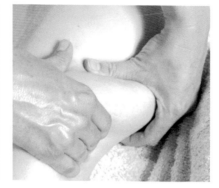
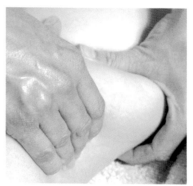

6) Wringing on the back of the thigh to cover the whole area twice

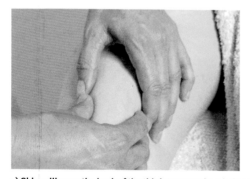
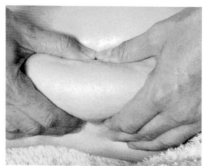
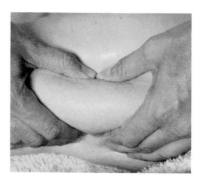

7) Skin rolling on the back of the thigh to cover the whole area twice

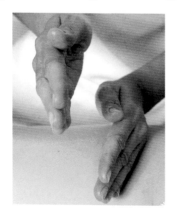
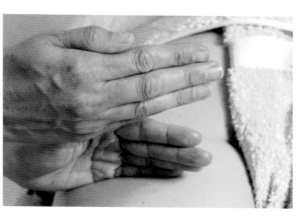

8) Hacking

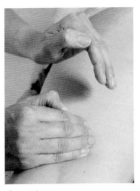 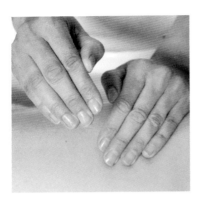 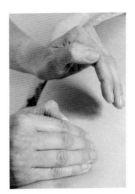

9) Cupping

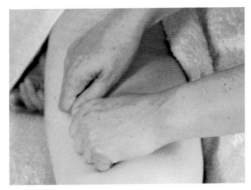 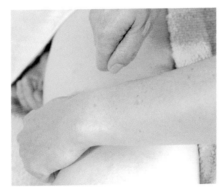

10) Beating

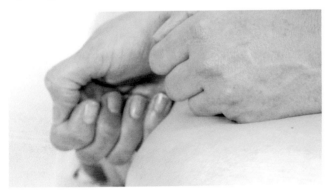 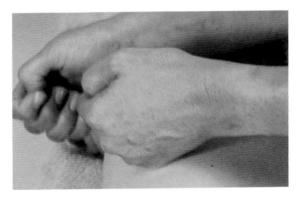

11) Pounding

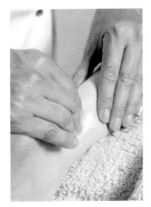 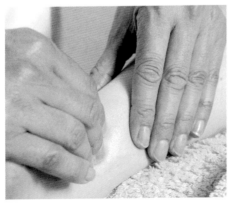 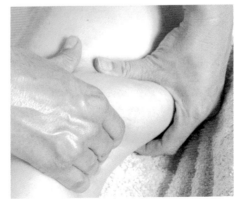

12) Picking up on the Achilles tendon

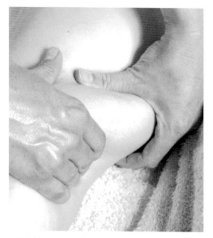

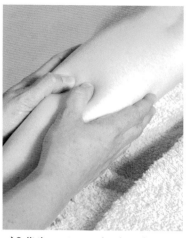

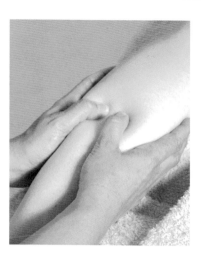

13) Picking up on the gastrocnemius and soleus twice

14) Split the gastrocnemius three times

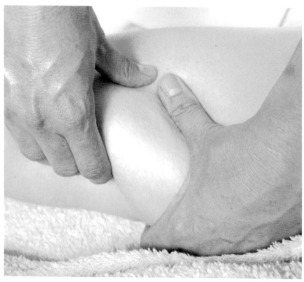

15) Wringing on the gastroc nemius and soleus twice

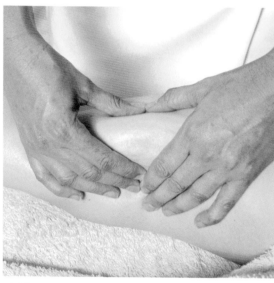

16) Skin rolling on the gastrocnemius and soleus twice

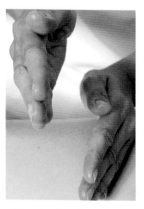

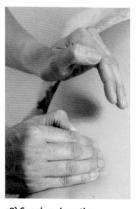

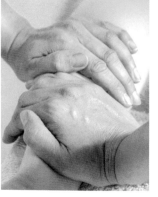

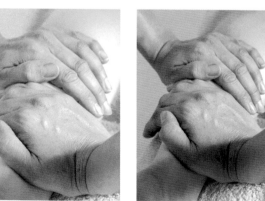

17) Hacking along the muscle fibres

18) Cupping along the muscles fibres

19) Effleurage the whole leg six times.

BACK   1) Effleurage to spread the oil

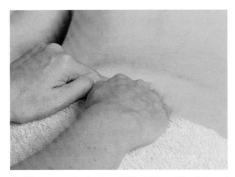 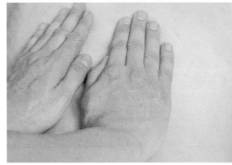

2) Effleurage twice in the middle (either side of the spine), twice slightly further out and twice to the sides of the body

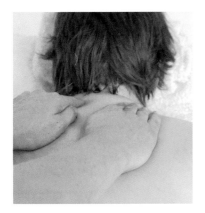 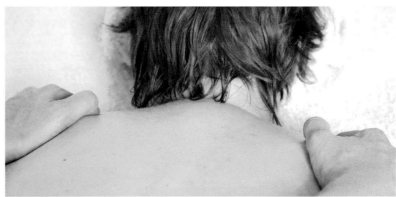

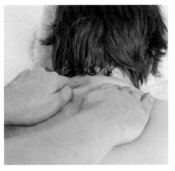 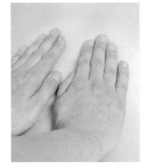

3) Palmar kneading six times in the same pattern   4) Alternate palmar kneading six times in the same pattern

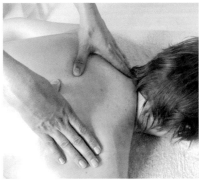 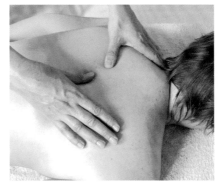 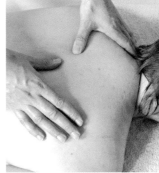

5) Thumb kneading to the rhomboids

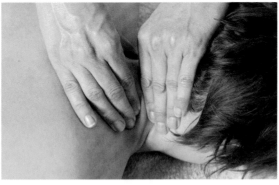
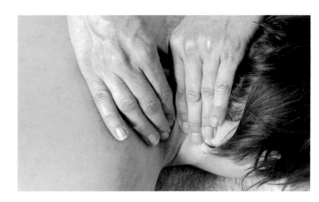

6) Kneading on the neck in the cervical area

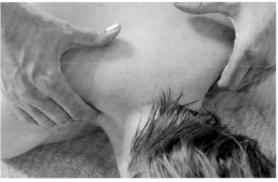
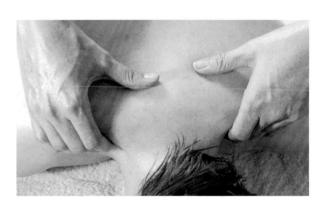

7) Skin rolling on the trapezius three times

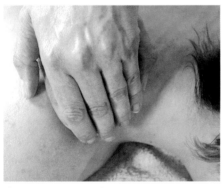
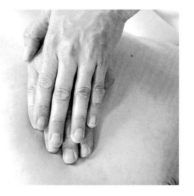

8) Figure of eight around the deltoid and scapula three times

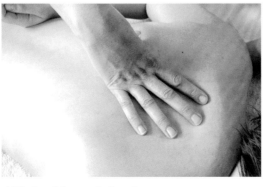
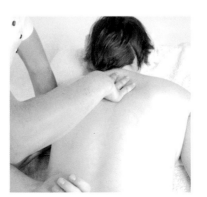

9) Winging of the scapula three times

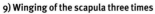

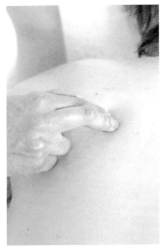

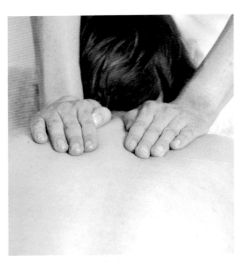

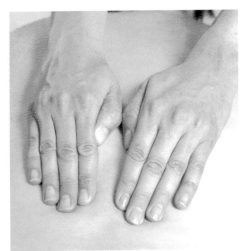

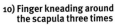

10) Finger kneading around
   the scapula three times

11) Reverse effleurage six times

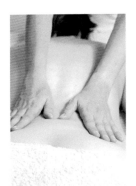

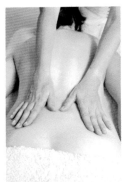

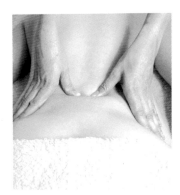

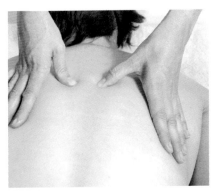

12) Thumb kneading up either side of the spine three times

13)   Thumb kneading the rhomboids three times.
14)   Picking up
15)   Wringing as before
16)   Skin rolling as before
17)   Hacking on the hips, upper arms and shoulders
18)   Cupping on the hips, upper arms and shoulders

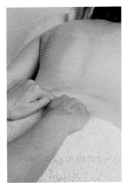

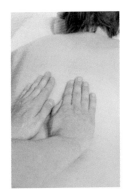

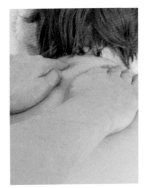

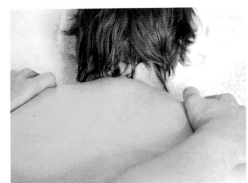

19) Effleurage twice in the middle (either side of the spine), twice slightly further out and twice to the sides of the body.

FACE MASSAGE: Spread the oil over the chest, shoulders, neck and face

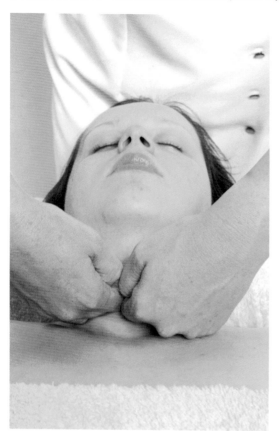

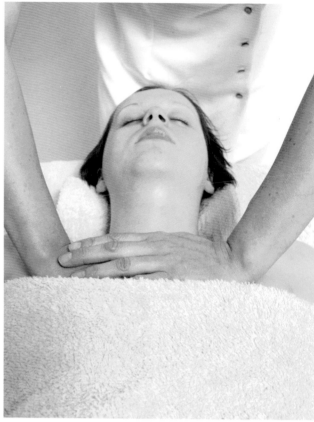

1) Effleurage the neck, chest and shoulders six times, covering the platysma, pectorals, deltoids and trapezius

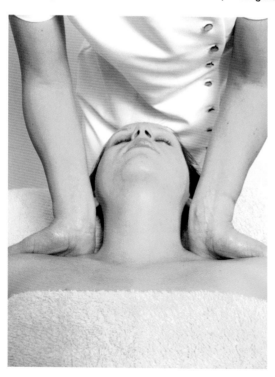

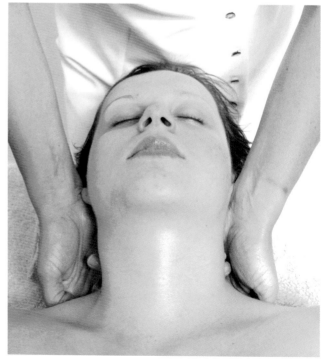

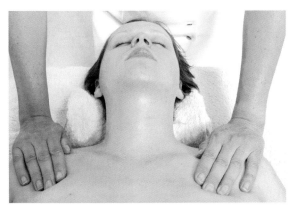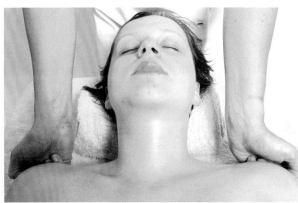

2) Rotations on the deltoids six times with an effleurage in between across the platysma, pectorals and trapezius muscles

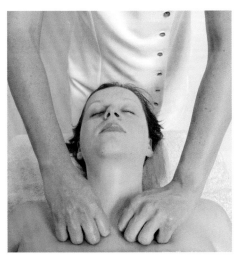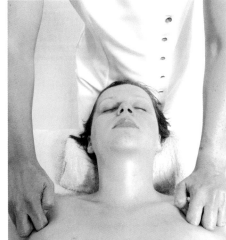

3) Knuckling across the pectorals, deltoids and trapezius six times

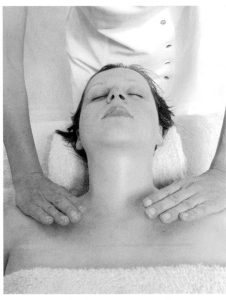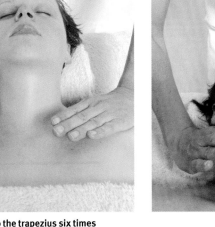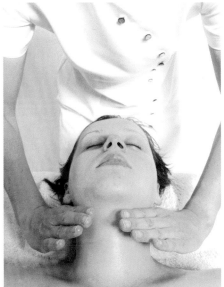

4) Thumb kneading to the trapezius six times

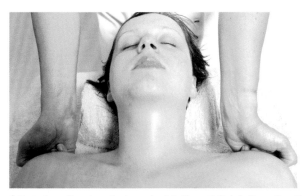
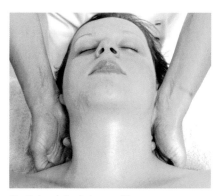

5) Finger kneading along the trapezius into the occipital six times. Turn the client's head slowly to one side

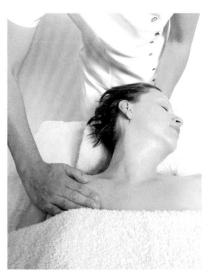
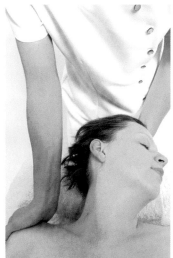
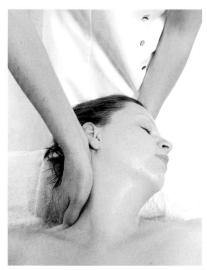

6) Six deep strokes up either side of the neck, using alternate hands, covering the sternocleido mastoid, the trapezius and platysma muscles

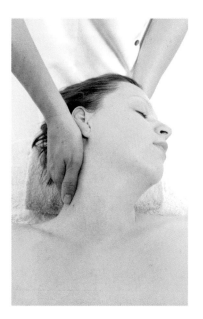
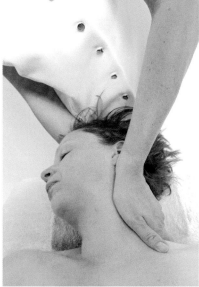
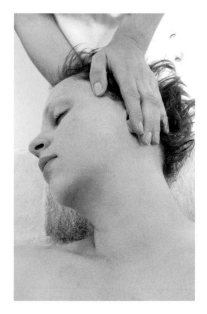

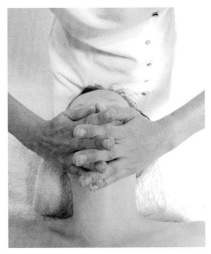
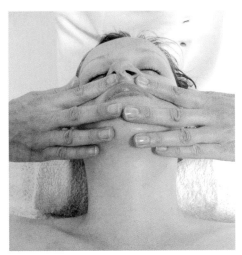
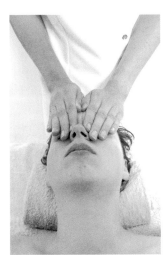

7) Three full face braces

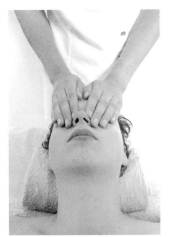
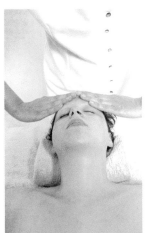
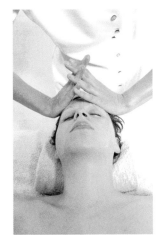
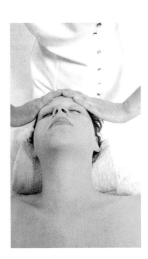

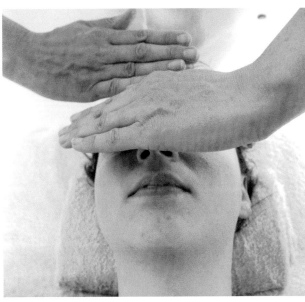
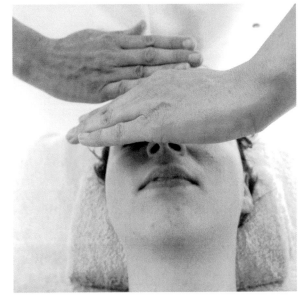

8) Stroke above the brow over the frontalis muscle twenty times

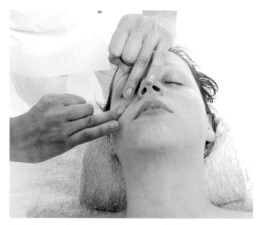
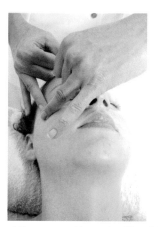
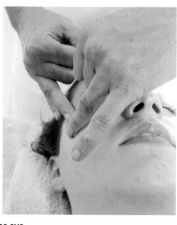

9) Half moon stroking under each eye six times

10) Alternate stroking at the sides of the eye

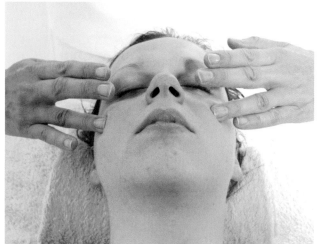
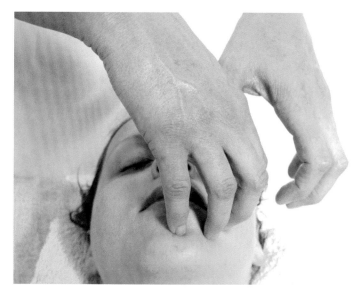

11) Full eye circles

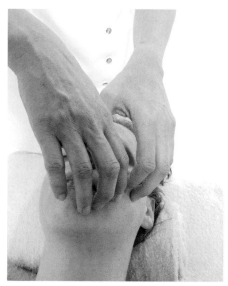

12) Tapping along the cheeks

13) Three full face braces (as stage 7)

14) Glide up to the scalp

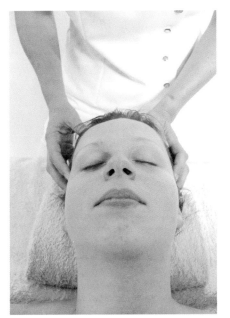

15) Stroke gently though the hair

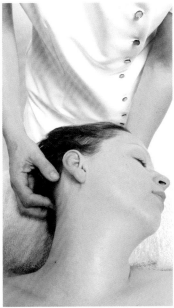

16) Petrissage

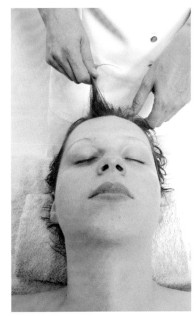

17) Gently pull on the hair

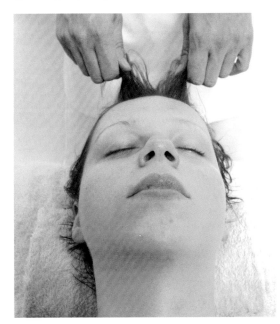

18) Knead around the edge of the ears

19) Effleurage the neck, chest and shoulders six times (as in stage 1)

20) Rotations on the deltoids six times (stage 2)

21) Knuckling across the pectorals, deltoids and trapezius six times (stage 3)

22) Thumb kneading to the trapezius six times (stage 4)

23) Finger kneading along the trapezius into the occipital six times (stage 5)

24) Three vibrations into the occipital.

ARMS

1) Effleurage to spread the oil

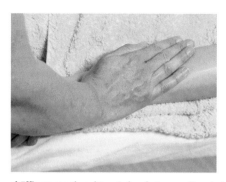 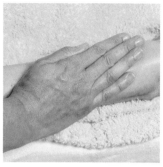 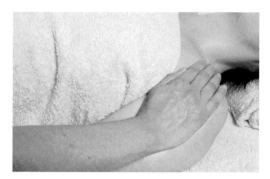

2) Effleurage using alternate hands to cover the whole arm six times

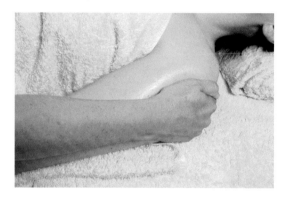 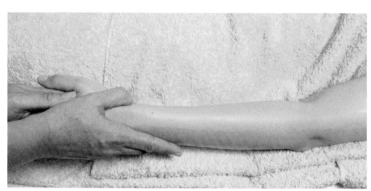

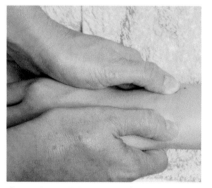 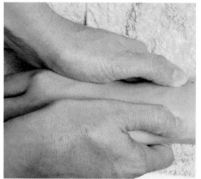 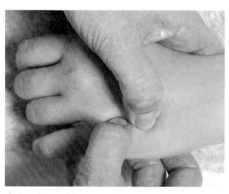

3) Knead around the carpals six times

4) Thumb knead between the metacarpals, little finger to thumb

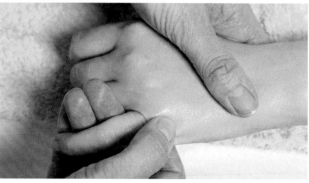 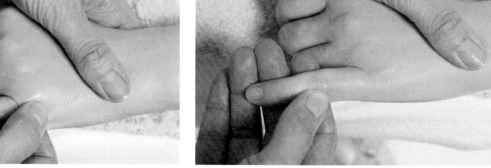

5) Thumb knead on the joints of the phalanges – little finger to thumb

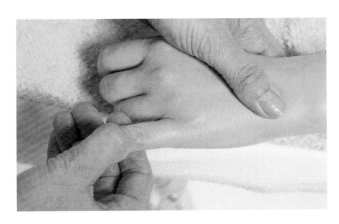

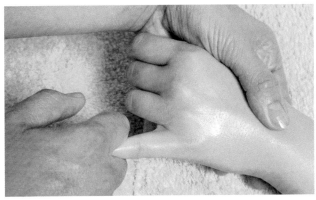

6) Gentle pulling on the fingers – little finger to thumb

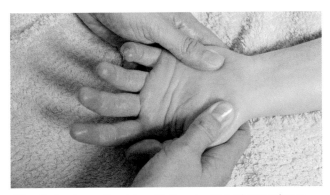

7) Turn the hand over – thumb knead to thenar and hypothenar eminence

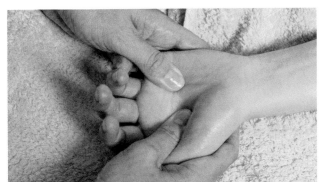

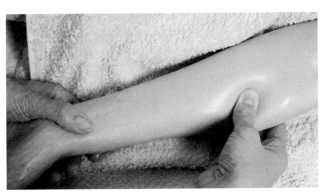

8) Kneading down from the elbow (superatrochlea lymph nodes) to the carpals

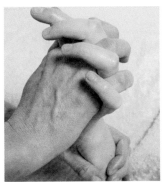
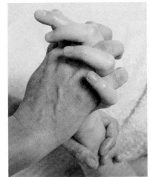

9) Rotate the hand clockwise three times very slowly

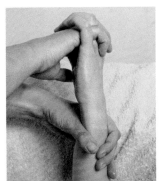

10) Reverse and rotate the hand anticlockwise three times very slowy

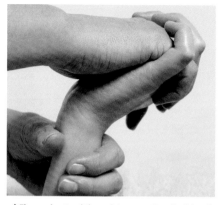
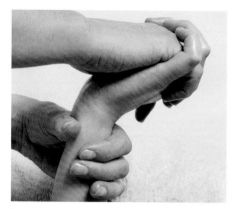

11) Flex and extend the wrist supporting the joint throughout the movement, twice each way

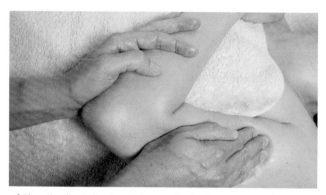
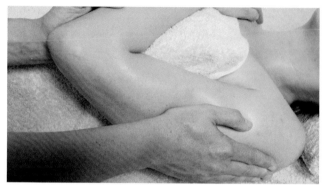

12) Place the client's hand on their opposite shoulder to open up the back of the arm. Palmar knead over the triceps six times

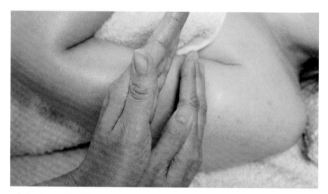
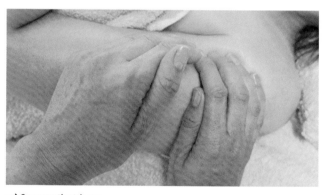

13) Hack over the triceps

14) Cup over the triceps

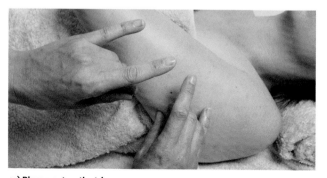
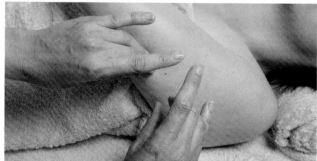

15) Pincement on the triceps

16) Effleurage using alternate hands to cover the whole arm six times (as in 2).

ABDOMEN

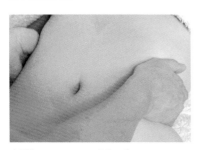

1) Effleurage to spread the oil

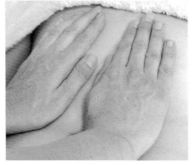

2) Effleurage six times, two to the centre, two moving out and two to the sides of the abdominal region

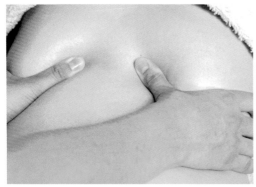

3) Six breathing movements

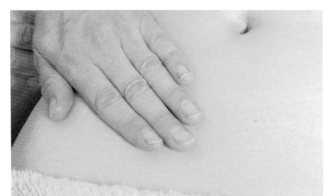

4) Pulling either side of the waist

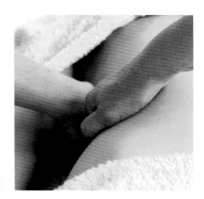

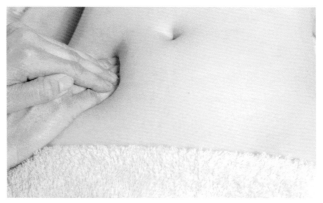

5) Circular effleurage, around the colon

6) Reinforced kneading around the colon

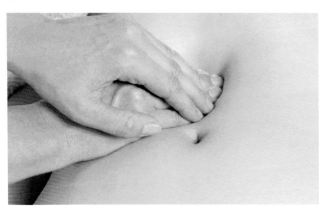

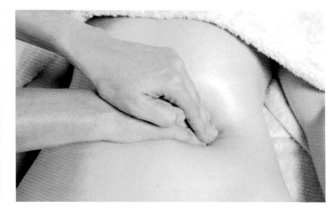

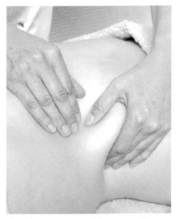
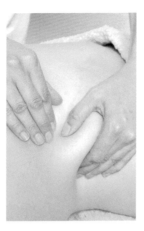

7) Picking up on the abdomen working in the shape of a W

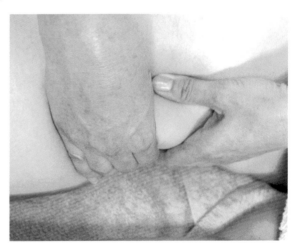

8) Wringing on the abdomen working in the shape of a W

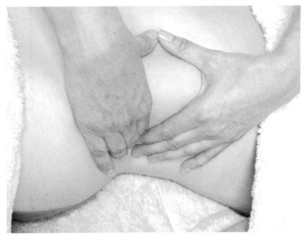

9) Skin rolling on the abdomen working in the shape of a W

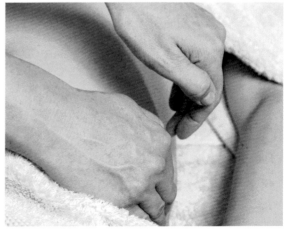

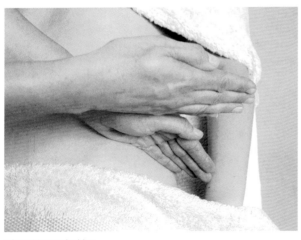

10) Hacking to the hips

11) Cupping on the hips

12) Effleurage six times, two to the centre, two moving out and two to the sides of the abdominal region (as in point 2)
13) Finish with deep pressure in the small of the back

FRONT OF LEGS

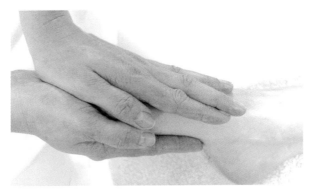

1) Effleurage to spread the oil

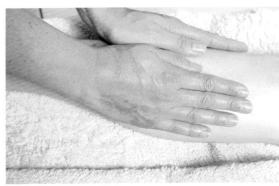

2) Effleurage the whole leg six times

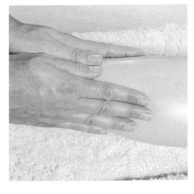

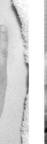

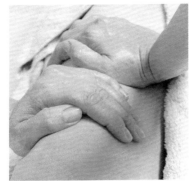

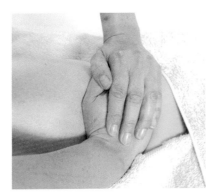

3) Palmar kneading to the top
of the thigh six times

4) Alternate palmar kneading to the top of the thigh six times

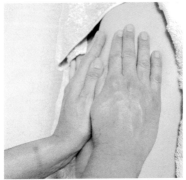

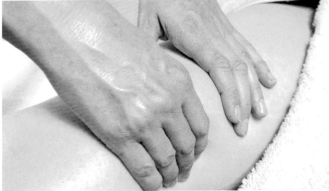

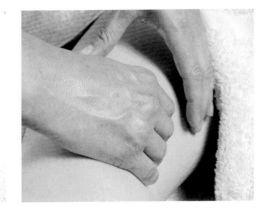

5) Picking up twice on the front of the thigh

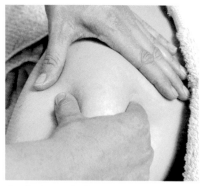

6) Wringing on the front of the thigh twice

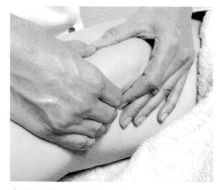

7) Skin rolling on the front of the thigh twice

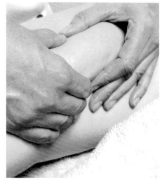

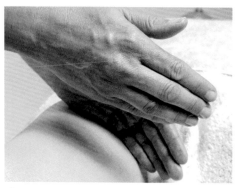

8) Hacking

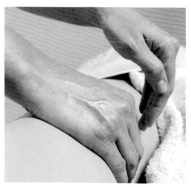

9) Cupping

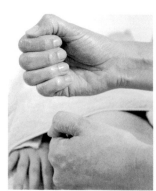

10) Beating

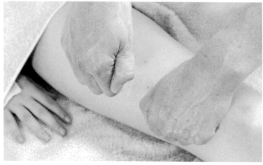

11) Pounding

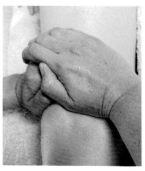

12) Effleurage up to and including patella six times

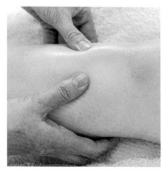

13) Thumb knead around patella three times

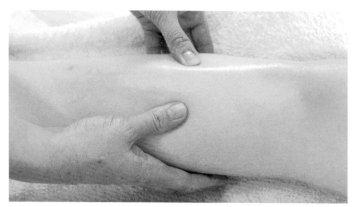

14) Knead either side of the tibia twice moving down to the tarsals

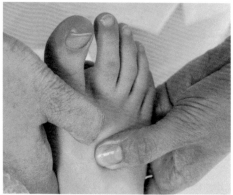

15) Thumb knead between the metatarsals, little toe to big toe

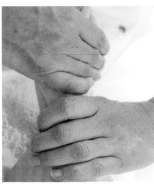

16) Full toe rotations (once each way, all the toes together)

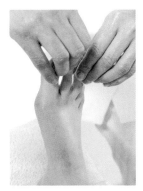

17) Picking on the toes

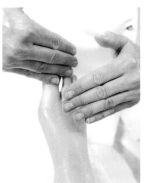

18) Whipping on the toes

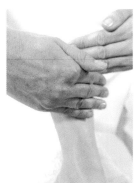

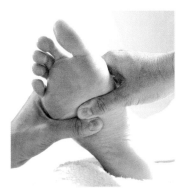

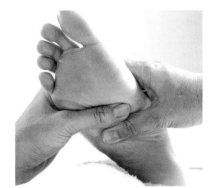

19) Cross frictions down the foot using the thumbs, then working back up

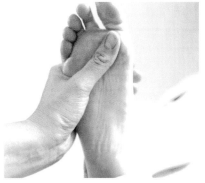

20) Flex and extend the foot, twice each way

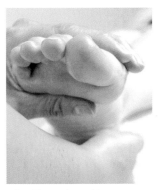

21) Ankle rotations whilst supporting the ankle joint, three times one way then reverse

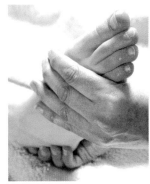

22) Effleurage the whole leg six times (as in point 2)

23) Cover the leg gently with the towel

24) Hold onto the client's feet through the towels

25) Energise with the palms of your hands on the client's feet

26) Move up the couch and place one hand on the client's abdomen on top of the towels and the other on the client's forehead

27) Then take your hands away from the client so slowly that they feel as though you are still touching them.

Example of client record

Client Consultation Form – Holistic

ITEC

College Name: A Sample
College Number: 1234
Learner Name: A Sample
Learner Number: 1234
Date: 01/1/11

Client Name: Mrs MB
Address: Derby

Profession: Management Accountant
Tel. No: **Day** 1234 56789
Eve 1234 56789

PERSONAL DETAILS

Age group: ☐ **Under 20** ☐ **20–30** ☐ **30–40** ☑ **40–50** ☐ **50–60** ☐ **60+**
Lifestyle: ☑ **Active** ☐ **Sedentary**
Last visit to the doctor: ☐ At least 6 months ago
GP Address: Derby
No. of children (if applicable): None
Date of last period (if applicable): 1/12/10

CONTRAINDICATIONS REQUIRING MEDICAL PERMISSION – in circumstances where medical permission cannot be obtained clients must give their informed consent in writing prior to treatment (select where/if appropriate):

☐ Pregnancy
☐ Cardiovascular conditions (thrombosis, phlebitis, hypertension, hypotension, heart conditions)
☐ Haemophilia
☐ Any condition already being treated by a GP or another complementary practitioner
☐ Medical oedema
☐ Osteoporosis
☐ Arthritis
☐ Nervous/Psychotic conditions
☐ Epilepsy
☐ Recent operations
☐ Asthma
☐ Diabetes
☐ Chemotherapy
☐ Chemotherapy
☐ Radiotherapy

☐ Any dysfunction of the nervous system (e.g. Multiple sclerosis, Parkinson's disease, Motor neurone disease)
☐ Bells Palsy
☐ Trapped/Pinched nerve (e.g. sciatica)
☐ Inflamed nerve
☐ Cancer
☐ Postural deformities
☐ Cervical spondylitis
☐ Spastic conditions
☐ Kidney infections
☐ Whiplash
☐ Slipped disc
☐ Undiagnosed pain
☐ When taking prescribed medication
☐ Acute rheumatism
☐ Medication causing thinning/inflammation of the skin
☐ Diagnosed scleroderma

CONTRAINDICTIONS THAT RESTRICT TREATMENT (select where/if appropriate):

☐ Fever
☐ Contagious or infectious diseases
☐ Under the influence of recreational drugs or alcohol
☐ Diarrhoea and vomiting
☐ Skin diseases
☐ Undiagnosed lumps and bumps
☐ Localised swelling
☐ Inflammation
☐ Varicose veins
☐ Pregnancy (abdomen)
☐ Cuts
☐ Bruises
☐ Abrasions
☐ Scar tissues (2 years for major operation and 6 months for a small scar)
☐ Sunburn
☐ Hormonal implants

☐ Menstruation (abdomen - first few days)
☐ Haematoma
☐ Hernia
☐ Recent fractures (minimum 3 months)
☐ Gastric ulcers
☐ After a heavy meal
☐ Conditions affecting the neck
☐ Any metal pins or plates
☐ Loss of skin sensation (test with tactile test)
☐ IUD (coil)
☐ Anaphylaxis
☐ Muscle fatigue
☐ Pacemaker
☐ Body piercing
☐ Excessive erythema
☐ Recent dermabrasion or chemical peels
☐ Recent IPL, laser and/or epilation

WRITTEN PERMISSION REQUIRED BY:

☐ GP/Specialist ☐ Informed consent
Either of which should be attached to the consultation form.

Example of client record (continued)

PERSONAL INFORMATION (select if/where appropriate):

Muscular/Skeletal problems: ☐ Back ☐ Aches/Pain ☐ Stiff joints ☐ Headaches

Digestive problems: ☐ Constipation ☐ Bloating ☐ Liver/Gall bladder ☐ Stomach

Circulation: ☐ Heart ☐ Blood pressure ☐ Fluid retention ☐ Tired legs ☐ Varicose veins
☑ Cellulite ☐ Kidney problems ☐ Cold hands and feet

Gynaecological: ☐ Irregular periods ☐ P.M.T ☐ Menopause ☐ H.R.T ☐ Pill ☐ Coil
Other:

Nervous system: ☐ Migraine ☐ Tension ☐ Stress ☐ Depression

Immune system: ☐ Prone to infections ☐ Sore throats ☐ Colds ☐ Chest ☐ Sinuses

Regular antibiotic/medication taken? ☐ Yes ☑ No
If yes, type and name of remedy

Herbal remedies taken? ☐ Yes ☑ No
If yes, which ones:

Ability to relax: ☐ Good ☑ Moderate ☐ Poor

Sleep patterns: ☑ Good ☐ Poor ☐ Average No. of hours 7

Do you see natural daylight in your workplace? ☑ Yes ☐ No

Do you work at a computer? ☑ Yes ☐ No If yes how many hours: 6-7

Do you eat regular meals? ☑ Yes ☐ No

Do you eat in a hurry? ☑ Yes ☐ No

Do you take any food/vitamin supplements? ☐ Yes ☑ No
If yes, type and name of supplement(s)

How many portions of each of these items does your diet contain per day?
Fresh fruit: 2 Fresh vegetables: 1 ☑ Protein Source of protein: Chicken, fish, cheese
Dairy produce: O Sweet things: 1 Added salt: O Added sugar: O

How many units of these drinks do you consume per day?
Tea: 1 Herbal: O Coffee: 5 Fruit juice: 2 Water: O Soft drinks: O Others: O

Do you suffer from food allergies? ☐ Yes ☑ No

Do you suffer from eating disorders? ☐ Bingeing ☐ Yes ☑ No
Overeating? ☐ Yes ☑ No Undereating? ☐ Yes ☑ No

Do you smoke? ☐ Yes ☑ No How many per day?

Do you drink alcohol? ☑ Yes ☐ No How many units per day? 1-2 glasses of wine with meals

Do you exercise? ☑ Yes ☐ No ☐ Occasional ☐ Irregular ☐ Regular
Types of exercise: Swimming, walking, cycling

What is your skin type? ☑ Dry ☐ Oily ☐ Normal ☐ Young ☐ Mature

Do you suffer/have you suffered from: ☐ Dermatitis ☐ Acne ☑ Eczema Small patches on her hands
☐ Psoriasis ☐ Allergies ☐ Hay Fever ☐ Asthma ☐ Skin cancer

TREATMENT (select where/if appropriate):

☑ Body Scrub ☑ Mechanical Massage (G5) ☑ Galvanism ☐ Vacuum suction
☐ Microcurrent ☐ Faradism ☑ Body Massage ☑ Body wrap ☐ Body mask

Example of client record (continued)

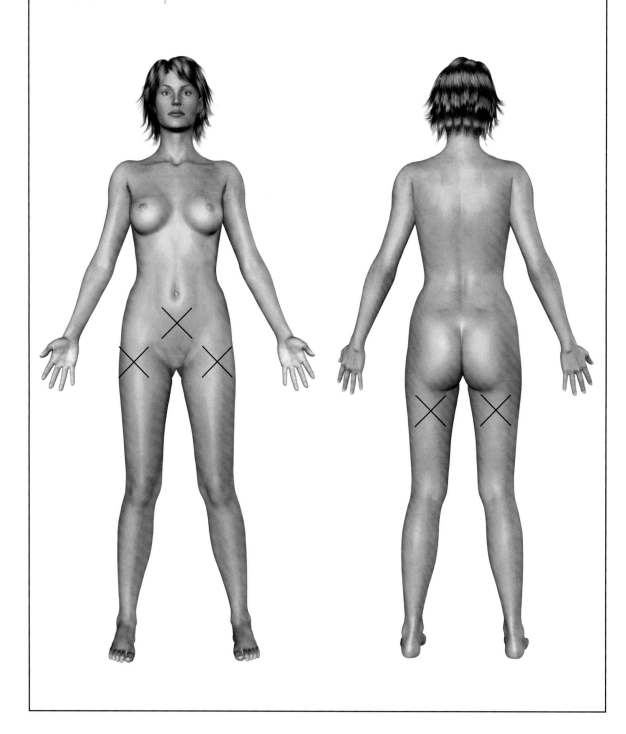

BODY ANALYSIS:

Height: *5ft 6ins*

Weight: *10st*

Body type/conditions: *Endomorph*

Postural conditions: *None*

Types of fat: *Cellulite on thighs, soft fat on abdomen*

Skin type/condition: *Dry*

Example of client record (continued)

MEASUREMENTS:
Upper chest (under the arms): 25"
Maximum chest: 34"
Below bust: 30"
Waist: 28"
Hips: 37"
Maximum buttocks (on hairline): 39"

Top of thigh: Right:21"   Left: 21"
1 inch/2cm above knee: R: 16" L: 16.5"
Maximum calf muscle: R: 13" L: 13"
Ankle: R: 9" L: 9"
Middle of upper arm: R: 11" L: 10.5"
Middle of lower arm: R: 10.5" L: 10"
Wrist: R: 6" L: 6"

MUSCLE TEST (select if/where appropriate):

Quadriceps:	☐ Excellent	☑ Good	☐ Average	☐ Poor
Hamstrings:	☐ Excellent	☑ Good	☐ Average	☐ Poor
Biceps:	☐ Excellent	☑ Good	☐ Average	☐ Poor
Triceps:	☐ Excellent	☑ Good	☐ Average	☐ Poor
Abdominal:	☐ Excellent	☑ Good	☐ Average	☐ Poor

TESTS
Nerve (tactile) sensitivity test: ☑ Yes ☐ No
Heat (thermal) sensitivity test: ☑ Yes ☐ No

EXERCISE ADVICE:
Target area abdominals and thighs:
- Short warm up (5 mins)
- sit ups – 10 reps
- diagonals situps10 reps,
- plank holding for 30 seconds and building up to a min
- Squats 10 reps
- Lunges 10 reps each side
Repeat all the above 3 times
- cools down(5 mins)

Treatment details:
Target - abdominal area and cellulite on the lower buttocks and outer thighs
Treatment plan;
- Body scrub – jojoba and apricot kernel
- Moisturising body wrap
- G5 with particular emphasis on the tapotement and petrissage heads
- Faradic on abdominal muscles– bi-phasic setting- 20 minutes.
- Galvanic - iontophoresis treatment on thighs - 10 minutes
- Swedish body massage using grape seed oil with particular emphasis on the problem areas – 45 minutes

Client Feedback:
The client was satisfied with the treatment and felt that her abdominal muscles had received a good work out. She found the galvanic treatment irritating but accepted that it should improve her cellulite. She enjoyed the massage and noticed that it had improved the texture of her skin.

After/Home care advice given:
- Advise the client to book a course of treatments –twice a week for a minimum of 6 weeks
- Avoid any heat treatments, including very hot showers and baths.
- Increase water intake
- Body brush daily particularly on the thighs
- Use daily moisturiser
- Use a specific anti-cell tie product on the thighs

Client's signature ....

Learners's signature ....

DON'T FORGET
TO LOGIN TO GAIN ACCESS TO YOUR **FREE** MULTI-MEDIA LEARNING RESOURCES

☐ **Over 40 minutes of instructional videos of all the key treatments**

☐ **Lesson plans and multiple choice and essay questions**

☐ **Interactive games and quizzes to help you to test your knowledge**

To login to use these resources visit
www.emspublishing.co.uk/spa and follow the onscreen instructions.

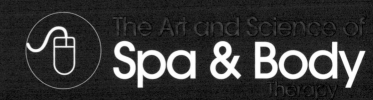

The Art and Science of
Spa & Body
Therapy

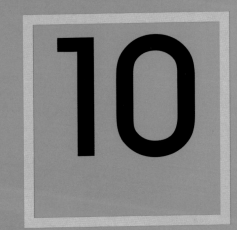

10

The science of electrical treatments

As therapists we are aiming to improve the overall condition of the skin and contours of the body. This sometimes requires a deeper, more intense treatment in order to maximise inch loss which may require the use of electrical equipment.
Effective, professional and safe practice requires us to understand something of the interactions and techniques we are employing, together with their effects and implications for the client and therapist.

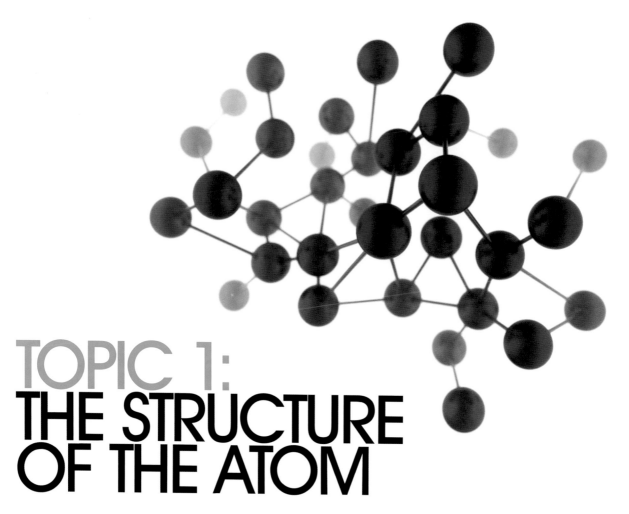

TOPIC 1:
THE STRUCTURE OF THE ATOM

The world around us (and including us) us is made up of a myriad of tiny particles, called atoms. These atoms are of a number of different types, or elements, such as carbon, iron, oxygen or hydrogen. The existence of atoms as one of the smallest building blocks of the physical world was first suggested by the ancient Greek, Democritus, but really became an accepted model when restated by Dalton in the nineteenth century.

An understanding of atoms, their structure and behaviour permits an understanding of many of the physical effects that we use or harness as beauty therapists. Atoms, combined together through chemical reactions to form molecules, make up the world around us, the cosmetic products we use and even our clients and ourselves. The atoms of different elements are constructed of different numbers of these particles and hence have different atomic weights. These are expressed relative to the mass of a carbon atom, which is set at twelve. On this scale, a hydrogen atom (the lightest atom) has a mass of one.

Smaller and smaller

Everything is composed of tiny particles called atoms, and they themselves are composed of smaller sub-atomic particles, called protons, neutrons and electrons.

The three particles vary in other ways besides

• DON'T FORGET

Watch the electrical treatment videos on the included CD-ROM.

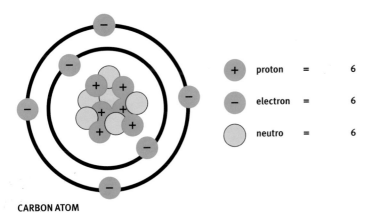

+ proton	=	6
− electron	=	6
○ neutro	=	6

CARBON ATOM

their mass. Neutrons, as their name implies, are electrically neutral. Protons, on the other hand, have a positive electrical charge. Each electron in the atom has a negative electrical charge of the same size as the positive charge on a proton. The positively charged protons, and negatively charged electrons are attracted together. In an atom, there are the same number of protons and electrons, leaving atoms electrically neutral overall.

Ions

If an atom loses or gains electrons, so that it no longer has an equal number of electrons and protons, then its overall electrical charge will no longer be zero and, in this state, it is called an ion. If it has gained electrons it will have become negatively charged overall, and is known as an anion, and if it has lost electrons (becoming positively charged), it will be known as a cation.

Just as we are made of many molecules, and molecules are made of a number of atoms, atoms themselves are made up of a number of smaller sub-atomic particles, called protons, neutrons and electrons.

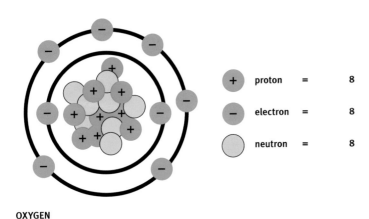

+ proton	=	8
− electron	=	8
○ neutron	=	8

OXYGEN

Sub-atomic particles

The protons and neutrons (which have similar masses very close to one) within an atom form a nucleus at its centre, about which the electrons (which have a relatively tiny mass) orbit. A hydrogen atom, which has a mass of one, will have one proton in its nucleus, with a single electron orbiting it.

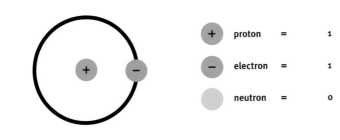

+ proton	=	1
− electron	=	1
○ neutron	=	0

HYDROGEN

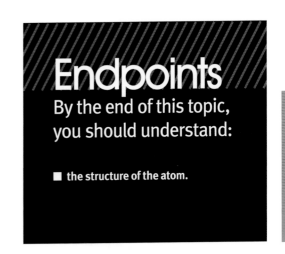

Endpoints
By the end of this topic, you should understand:

■ the structure of the atom.

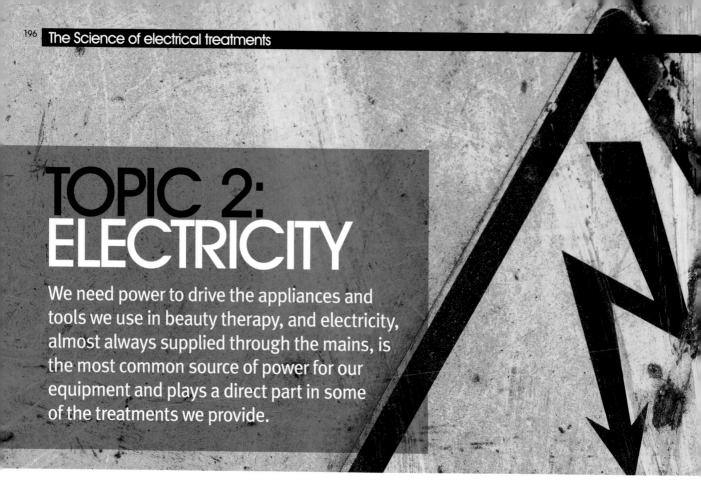

TOPIC 2: ELECTRICITY

We need power to drive the appliances and tools we use in beauty therapy, and electricity, almost always supplied through the mains, is the most common source of power for our equipment and plays a direct part in some of the treatments we provide.

THE MEASUREMENT OF ELECTRICITY

An electrical current (measured in Amperes, or Amps, symbol A) is a flow of electrons through a conductor such as a wire. This flow of electrons is caused by an applied potential difference (measured in Volts, symbol V) or voltage. A simple way to think of this is as the voltage representing the pressure on the water in a hosepipe, and the current representing the flow of water through the pipe.

The voltage and current are related. For the same piece of wire, a higher voltage results in a higher current, and vice versa – much as turning up the tap to a hosepipe results in a greater flow of water through it. The relationship between voltage and current is expressed through Ohm's law, which introduces another factor – resistance – to describe the characteristics of the conductor. To continue our hosepipe analogy, if we replace our normal hosepipe with a very narrow one, less water will flow through for the same setting on the tap. The resistance of a conductor is a measure of its resistance to current flowing through it. For the same voltage, a higher resistance allows less current to flow than a lower resistance.

Ohm's law is very simple:

Voltage = Current x Resistance or V = I x R

TYPES OF ELECTRIC CURRENT

An alternating current (AC) flows in one direction, then the other, continually reversing, much as the flow of water in waves on a beach flows back and forth. A direct current (DC) flows in one direction only, as the water in a river flows in one direction only. The current that flows from a mains socket into an appliance is an alternating current – you will see the inputs to equipment marked with the voltage they accept and that it is AC.

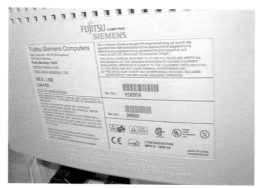

THE DANGERS OF ELECTRICAL CURRENTS

Electrical currents can be dangerous if not used correctly. The electrical shock from a malfunctioning piece of salon equipment can be as lethal as a lightning strike, and so the proper selection, usage, maintenance and testing of electrical equipment is essential.

The physiological risks of electrical currents

The physical damage caused by electrical currents falls into three main areas – burns, effects on the heart and neurological system.

1. **Burns.** As the current tries to flow through the body, the resistance of the body causes tissues to heat up. This can cause severe burns deep in the body, especially at higher voltages with sources that can provide high currents.

2. **The heart.** The effect of an electrical shock on the heart can cause ventricullar fibrillation – disrupting the contraction of the muscles of the heart – which is usually lethal. Even at a low voltage such as that supplied by the mains (240v AC), ventricular fibrillation may be induced in the heart after a fraction of a second of a current as low as a twentieth of an Ampere travelling through the chest. A higher current is needed if the voltage is DC.

3. **Effects on the neurological system.** An electric shock can affect the operation of the nervous system, affecting the heart and lungs in particular. If the shock runs through the head, a large enough current can cause unconsciousness and death.

THE EFFECTS OF THERAPEUTIC ELECTRICAL CURRENTS ON BODY TISSUES

1. Faradic treatments

Faradic treatments are used to tone muscles and firm facial contours. In a Faradic treatment a low-voltage direct current is applied under the control of the therapist, via an electrode placed on the skin on the motor point of the muscle that requires stimulation. This causes the muscle to contract (stimulation period) and relax (stimulation interval).

2. Microcurrent treatments

Microcurrent treatments use low-frequency (1 to 20 Hz) microcurrents (micro-amps) to re-educate muscle tone, shortening muscle fibres where they lack tone. The low current is undetectable to the client. The stimulation should improve the appearance of the skin by stimulating and tightening the facial and body muscles and through increasing blood flow to the area. It is frequently used as an anti-ageing treatment and is often referred to as the 'face lift without the knife'.

3. Modified direct current

Modified direct current treatments use a varying, but still direct, current to stimulate the muscles. An active substance is applied to the skin. The electrode carrying the same charge as the active substance will repel the active substance into the skin. The choice of treatment depends on the polarity of the active substance so it is vital the manufacturer's instructions are always adhered to – the positively charged electrode will repel a positively charged substance, and the negatively charged electrode will repel a negatively charged one. The rate of iontophoretic transport is affected by several factors including skin pH, active ingredient concentration, current, voltage, time applied and skin resistance.

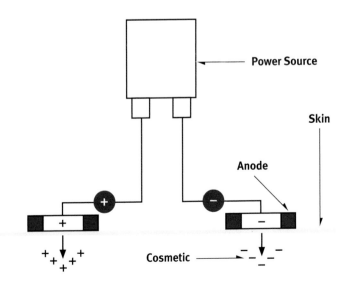

The iontophoretic circuit

TRANSFORMERS

We may sometimes need a higher or lower voltage than the 240V available from the mains supply. To achieve this, salon equipment incorporates a device called a transformer. The transformer is a device that can increase or decrease the voltage of an AC supply. It cannot change the voltage of a DC supply, nor can it affect the frequency of an AC one.

A transformer that has a higher output voltage than input voltage is called a step-up transformer, and one that has a lower output than input voltage is called a step-down transformer. A transformer is to be found inside the power supply of almost every piece of electrical equipment used by the therapist, where it is used to reduce the voltage of the incoming mains supply to a level more suitable for use in the equipment, machines that use an alternating current, such as high-frequency machines will also include one.

RECTIFIERS

We saw earlier that there are two types of current: alternating and direct. We may need to convert AC current, which is supplied in the mains supply, to DC. To do this we use a device called a rectifier. In most cases, you will never see a rectifier – it will be a component contained within the power supply of a piece of equipment. To covert AC current to DC current, we need to stop it flowing back and forth, and to make it flow in one direction only. This is the function of the rectifier. The rectifier itself contains electronic components called diodes, which only allow current to flow in one direction – they are like doors which only open in one direction.

Endpoints

By the end of this topic, you should understand:

- the measurement of electricity
- the different types of current used in beauty therapy
- the possible risks involved and the effects of currents on body tissue
- the function of a transformer
- the function of a rectifier.

Primary Winding
Np turns

Secondary Winding
N8 turns

Primary Current
1p

Primary Voltage
1/p

Secondary
Current 1s

Secondary
Voltage 1/s

TOPIC 3: ELECTROMAGNETIC RADIATION AND BEAUTY THERAPY

Light, radio waves, ultra violet and infra-red are all types of electromagnetic radiation. We spend our lives bathed in electromagnetic radiation from a variety of natural and artificial sources and, in our work as beauty therapists, we harness the effects of various types of electromagnetic radiation on the body in order to help our clients.

The spectrum of electromagnetic radiation runs across a range of frequencies and wavelengths, extending above and below the visible portion of the spectrum. The visible portion of the spectrum is determined by the nature of our own eyes — much as the range of sounds we can hear depends on the nature of our ears. With sound there are sounds pitched above and below the range of human senses that we cannot hear. Just as sounds range in frequency across a wide spectrum, so does electromagnetic radiation range above and below the range of our own senses, extending down in frequency from the red end of the visible part of the spectrum to infra-red radiation and then down further to radio waves, and up in frequency from the violet end of the visible spectrum into ultra violet light, and then upwards towards X-rays, gammarays and cosmic rays.

However, as anyone who has spent too long on the beach can testify, electromagnetic radiation (in this case the ultra violet light in sunlight) can have unpleasant effects on the skin. Professionalism, safety and efficiency therefore require that we understand the nature, behaviour and effects of the various different types of electromagnetic radiation.

THE STRUCTURE OF THE ELECTROMAGNETIC SPECTRUM

The light in which we see our world is made up of a mixture of coloured light of different wavelengths – which we can see separated out into a spectrum when we see a rainbow, or look at the light reflected from the underside of a CD.

Different types of electromagnetic radiation

Radiation from the electromagnetic spectrum is all around us, from the radio waves generated by our mobile phones, to the colours of sunlight and up to and beyond the UV light from sunbeds.

Just as a sound can be high or low-pitched, electromagnetic radiation can be high or low frequency. The effect a sound has on us varies with both the pitch (or frequency) and the volume (or intensity). A really high-pitched whining sound might make our teeth stand on edge, and a very low frequency sound from something like ferry-boat engines can make our stomachs churn. Sound of intense volume endured night after night when clubbing can physically damage our ears. Just as sound waves can physically affect our bodies, so can electromagnetic radiation. Just as the effects of sound waves on our body depend on the frequency, intensity and length of exposure to the sound, so do the effects of electromagnetic radiation.

In beauty therapy, we make use of electromagnetic radiation in the infra-red region of the spectrum (with a wavelength of 4000 to 1000 nm) and in the ultra violet region (from around 100 nm to 400 nm).

THE EFFECTS OF ELECTROMAGNETIC RADIATION ON BODY TISSUES

Just as a sound can be loud or soft, electromagnetic radiation can be more or less intense – such as from a bright or dim light.

INFRA-RED RADIATION IN BEAUTY THERAPY

Beauty therapy makes use of two types:
1. **Infrared (4000 nm wavelength)**
2. **Radiant heat (1000 nm).**

An infra-red lamp uses an electrical filament to heat a clay element inside a focusing reflector until it emits radiation. The radiation is invisible, and the clay element does not glow when hot. The lamp will therefore be fitted with a guard to protect against touching the hot element.

Infra-red lamps are used for heating the skin (which must be clean and grease-free) before treatment, and exposures should not last longer

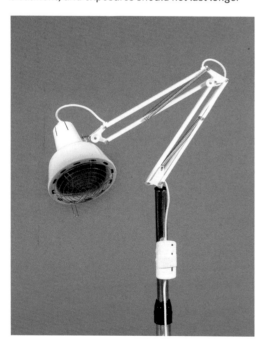

than ten minutes to prevent burning of the skin. The rays themselves do not penetrate deeply into the skin, but generate heat that causes vasodilation and increases blood and lymph flow. The radiation can damage the eye, causing cataracts, and so goggles should be worn, or eyes covered with damp cotton wool pads.

Lamps that produce radiant heat are now far more common in salon use. The lamp looks like a large light bulb, and contains a filament that emits small amounts of visible and ultra violet light in addition to infra-red heat. This is filtered by the characteristic red glass filter on the end of the lamp to ensure that no UV light reaches the client, only red and IR light.

Radiant heat lamps warm up more quickly than infrared lamps, but still become very hot in use. The lamp must not be allowed to touch and burn the skin, and care should be taken not to knock the lamp or splash fluids on it when it is hot, as this may cause it to shatter.

Because of the vasodilatory effect of infra red, it is contraindicated for clients with conditions such as broken capillaries and high colour or hyper-sensitive skins.

ULTRA VIOLET RADIATION IN BEAUTY THERAPY

As well as using infra red radiation in beauty therapy, we use electromagnetic radiation from beyond the other end of the visible spectrum. This is ultra violet (or UV) light, and is an invisible part of the spectrum that is higher in frequency than the violet end of the visible spectrum. UV light is classified into three types based on its wavelength (these figures may vary slightly):

Ultra violet light makes up about 5% of the radiation from the sun. In therapeutic use, it is generated in UV lamps containing mercury vapour. This may be at low pressure in the familiar tubes (LPMV), or high pressure (HPMV) in bulb-shaped lamps.

LPMV tubes produced almost entirely UVA light, with less than 1% UVB and almost no UVC. HPMV tubes produce all types of UV light, but reduce UVB and UVC levels to those of LPMV tubes by use of a filter that absorbs the unwanted radiation.

UV light is used in sunbeds, canopies and cubicles to produce a cosmetic tan. The

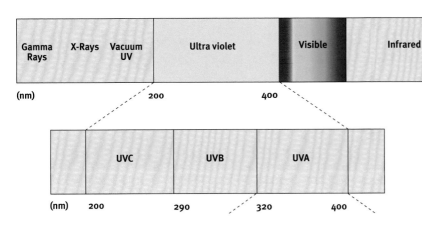

| Gamma Rays | X-Rays | Vacuum UV | Ultra violet | Visible | Infrared | Radio Waves |

(nm)   200   400

| UVC | UVB | UVA |

(nm)   200   290   320   400

Different types of electromagnetic radiation
Radiation from the electromagnetic spectrum is all around us, from the radio waves generated by our mobile phones, to the colours of sunlight and up to and beyond the UV light from sunbeds.

tanning response, which is due to the activity of melanocytes in the epidermis and oxidation and redistribution of existing melanin, begins during the exposure to UV radiation, is highest immediately after the treatment finishes, and will fade within an hour after exposure. The tanning effect will not provide protection for the skin against natural UV radiation. Tanning of any form is detrimental to all skin types, producing premature ageing, sun damage and possible skin cancers.

The different types of UV light penetrate to different depths in the skin, reaching different layers as they do so.

PENETRATION OF DIFFERENT UV WAVELENGTHS

Why is the inverse square law important to therapists? As the intensity reduces by a factor of four if you double the distance, this means that if you halve the distance between a client and a lamp you quadruple the intensity of the radiation on their skin. For the therapist, this is critically important when calculating safe and effective exposure times for their clients.

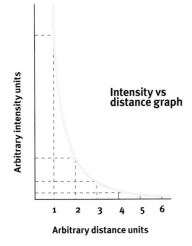

Intensity vs distance graph

Arbitrary intensity units

1   2   3   4   5   6

Arbitrary distance units

THE INVERSE SQUARE LAW

The closer we are to a heater, the hotter it feels, the closer we are to a lamp, the brighter it appears. The intensity of the radiation we feel from the source increases as we move closer to it, and reduces as we move further away. The radiation from a source (lamp, UV tube, etc.) escapes in all directions, spreading out as it does so. As you can see in the diagram, the amount of radiation that passes through an area of one square centimetre at a distance of one metre is the same as that passing through an area of four square centimetres at a distance of two metres. So the energy per square centimetre (or intensity) is reduced by a factor of four if the distance doubles.

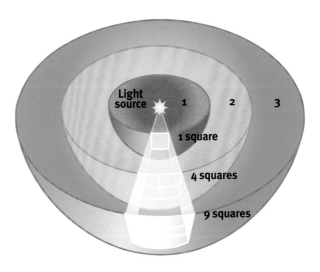

The intensity of the radiation is inversely proportional to the square of the distance from the source of the radiation – hence the name inverse square law.

THE LINK BETWEEN DISTANCE, INTENSITY AND EXPOSURE TIMES

The intensity of rays varies inversely with the square of the distance from the lamp. Thus, the intensity of radiation from the same lamp at 30cm is four times that at 60cm and eleven times that at one metre, so a one minute exposure at 30cm distance is the equivalent of four minutes at 60cm and approximately eleven minutes at one metre.

Safety

Always remember that halving the distance between a client and a light source has the same effect as quadrupling the time they are exposed. Remember to base distances on the closest part of the client to the lamp.

Endpoints

By the end of this topic, you should understand:

- the structure of the electromagnetic spectrum
- the effects of electromagnetic radiation on body tissues
- the uses of infra red radiation in beauty therapy
- the uses of ultra violet radiation in beauty therapy
- the inverse square law
- the link between distance, intensity and exposure times.

TOPIC 4:
ELECTRICITY, SAFETY AND PROFESSIONALS

Re-read Chapter 1, to remind yourself about general but essential health and safety precautions, and about your and the salon's liability when dealing with the general public.

Both the employer and employee have duties towards health, safety and welfare of employees, and health and safety in the workplace. Failure in these duties may result in criminal liability and claims for damages, as well as serious consequences for people's health.

For the employer, the duties which relate to using electrical equipment include:

- **providing and maintaining:**
  - **safe systems at work**
  - **a safe work place**
  - **safe access and exits to the work place**
- **ensuring the safe handling, use and storage of substances and equipment**
- **providing the necessary information, instruction, training and supervision for health and safety.**

  For the employee, these duties include:
- **taking reasonable care of themselves, their clients or other staff for whom they are responsible**
- **not intentionally or recklessly misusing anything provided for health, safety or welfare.**

Anyone operating or owning electrical equipment used in a spa or salon should have:

- **every piece of electrical equipment tested at least once a year by a qualified electrician**
- **keep a written record of all tests which can be inspected**
- **regular inspections to detect simple faults, such as frayed cables or cracked plugs**

• KEY POINT

The function of the fuse is to prevent an appliance drawing an excessively high current.

- **a system of reporting and clearly marking faulty equipment and taking it out of use until it is repaired.**

This means that, as a therapist, you are responsible for the equipment you use.

EQUIPMENT CHECKLIST

- **Check that it is safe.**
- **Keep equipment in good condition.**
- **Alert your salon to any equipment that needs attention.**
- **Keep careful records.**
- **Only use electrical equipment that you have been trained to use.**
- **Do not use any equipment you think might be unsafe.**
- **Use equipment according to instructions.**
- **Take all necessary safety precautions.**
- **Your salon should provide all the necessary additional training in the use of their specific electrical equipment and in the safety procedures.**

FUSES

If an electrical appliance should fail, it is possible that it will fail in such a way as to draw a very heavy current from the mains supply. This current, converted to heat inside the equipment, may generate enough heat to cause a fire.

In order to prevent this happening, electrical appliances are fitted with fuses. A fuse consists of a small glass or ceramic tube with metal caps or contacts at each end.

Inside the body of the fuse, between the end

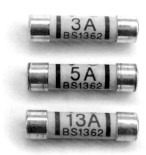

caps, is connected a piece of wire. The wire is designed, through thickness, electrical resistance, etc to heat up enough to melt when the current flowing through it reaches a certain limit. In this way, if the appliance that the fuse is protecting fails and begins to draw too much current, the wire inside the fuse will heat up and melt, thereby cutting off the supply of power to the equipment. In a glass bodied fuse when this has happened you can see that the wire inside is now broken. A ceramic-bodied fuse may show discolouration due to the heat generated when the wire inside melts.

Choosing the right fuse rating

For the greatest degree of protection, we need the fuse to blow at a current loading just over the normal current drawn by a correctly-working appliance. As different appliances will have different power-ratings, and hence draw different amounts of current when working correctly, the correct fuse rating will also vary. To allow for this, fuses are available in a range of ratings.

To decide what value of fuse to use, consult the appliance documentation, or look for information on the appliance itself. Do not assume that the fuse that has failed was of the correct rating – it may have been replaced with the wrong one by someone else.

If you know the power consumption of the appliance in watts, then you can calculate a suitable value for the fuse from the equation:

Current = Power/Voltage

For example mains voltage in the UK is 240 volts, a 700 watt appliance will draw 700/250 (or 2.8) amps of current. This is just less than a 3A fuse, and so a 3A fuse should be selected. Similarly we would use a:

• KEY POINT

Fuses come in 3A, 5A and 13A ratings. Use the right value – the fuse is there to protect you and your clients.

- 5 amp fuse with an appliance between 750 and 1000 watts
- 13 amp fuse for appliances between 1000 and 3000 watts

If the fuse blows repeatedly:
- do not replace it with a higher value
- disconnect the equipment and get it checked by a suitably qualified electrician.

CONTRAINDICATIONS AND SENSITIVITY TESTS FOR ELECTRICAL TREATMENTS

Before undertaking any treatment with a client, the therapist should always ensure the safety of the client and appropriateness of the treatment. See Chapter 3 for the contraindications that apply generally to all skin treatments. In addition, for electrical treatments, specific contraindications include:

- **heart disease – a weak heart may not be able to cope with the increased blood flow stimulated by the electrical current**
- **hypersensitive skin –**
- **increased circulation may cause irritation and worsening of broken capillaries**
- **epilepsy – electrical treatment may cause an epileptic episode**
- **pregnancy – do not apply an electric current through the body**
- **diabetes – due to loss of skin sensation and bruising**
- **metal pins and plates – loss of skin sensation (see below for tactile and thermal sensitivity tests)**
- **cute rheumatism**
- **osteoporosis**
- **trapped, pinched nerve**
- **pace makers**
- **body/face piercing.**

In addition to consideration of general and treatment specific contraindications, appropriate sensitivity tests should be performed. The purpose of sensitivity tests is to ensure that the client has normal, unimpaired sensitivity to stimuli, such as heat, pressure, etc, that provide warning against overexposure to the effects of some treatments. For electrical treatments, there are two important sensitivity tests that should be performed.

Nerve (tactile) sensitivity test

Before using an electrical treatment that stimulates the muscles, such as the faradic treatment, you must make sure that your client's sensory nerves are responding. Failure to do so could result in damaged facial muscles caused by the use of too high a current.

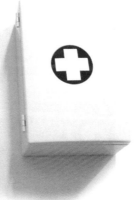

1. Ask your client to close their eyes.
2. Take a sharp object, such as an orange wood stick (rough), and then a soft object, such as cotton wool (smooth), and place them alternately on your client's skin.
3. Ask your client to say which is the rough and which is the smooth object.
   – If your client can tell the difference, they have good sensitivity and you can proceed with the treatment.
   – If your client cannot tell the difference, do not proceed; the treatment is then contraindicated.

Thermal sensitivity test

Before using an electrical heat treatment, such as infra red, you must make sure that your client's skin can differentiate between hot and cold sensations.

1. Fill two test tubes – one with hot water and one with cold water.
2. Place the test tubes alternately against your client's skin.
3. Ask your client to say which is the hot tube and which is the cold. If your client can feel the sensation of heat, and can tell the difference between the tubes, then you can proceed with the treatment. If your client cannot feel the difference, especially the feel of the hot tube, the treatment is contraindicated.

ELECTRICAL TREATMENTS AND FIRST AID

Because of the nature of electrical equipment which may, in an accident, cause either the therapist or the client to suffer electrical shock, burns or general shock, it is essential that you understand the guide to basic first aid and emergency procedure contained in Chapter 1. A therapist cannot administer first aid unless they are qualified to do so. However, it is very useful to know what to do, and you may consider taking a first aid qualification.

FIRST AID

A therapist should not give first aid unless qualified to do so, but should know the procedure for obtaining first aid.

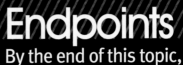

Endpoints
By the end of this topic, you should understand:

- the Health and Safety at Work Act 1974
- the Electricity at Work Act 1992
- fuses
- the correct wiring of a mains plug
- sensitivity tests for electrical treatments
- electrical treatments and first aid.

TOPIC 5: FARADIC TREATMENTS

Faradism is known as passive exercise as it exercises the muscles by passing an electrical current through them without any conscious effort of the client. The current causes the muscle to contract in the 'stimulating' period and relax in the stimulation interval to prevent muscle fatigue. Faradism is especially beneficial to atrophised muscles and loss of muscle tone It improves the general contours of the body.

THE EFFECTS OF FARADIC TREATMENTS

Faradism is used to:

- **improve muscle tone, by tightening and firming sagging muscles, enhancing and defining muscle tones**
- **increases local blood circulation and metabolism, bringing nourishment to the skin**
- **refine fine lines by improving facial and body contours**
- **stimulate nerve endings**
- **re-educate muscles that have been inactive**
- **increase blood and lymph flow, removing toxins and waste**
- **increase the energy-producing chemical ATP.**

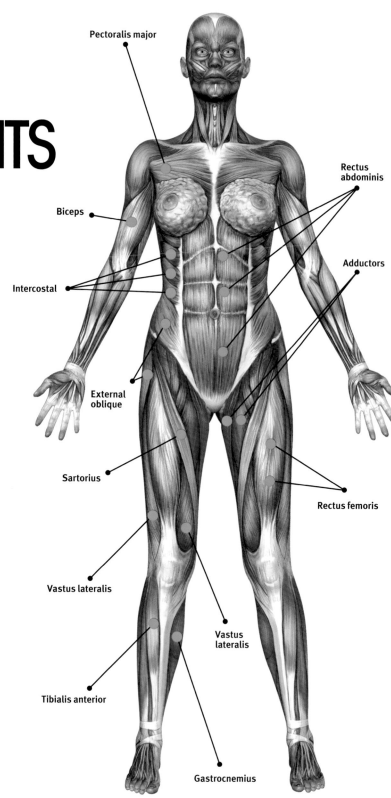

Pectoralis major

Rectus abdominis

Biceps

Adductors

Intercostal

External oblique

Sartorius

Rectus femoris

Vastus lateralis

Vastus lateralis

Tibialis anterior

Gastrocnemius

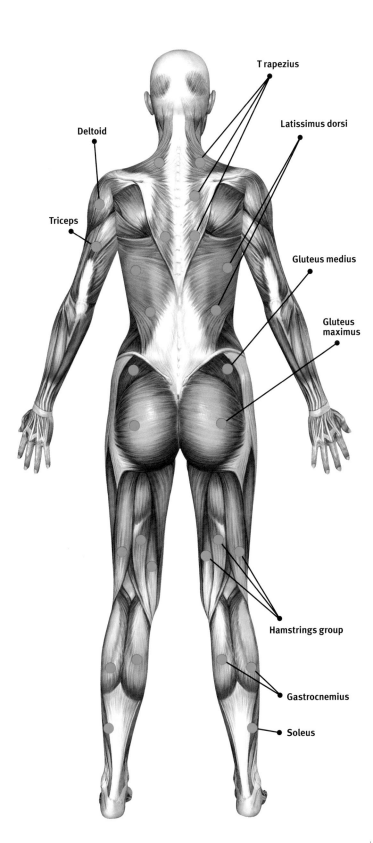

Trapezius

Latissimus dorsi

Deltoid

Triceps

Gluteus medius

Gluteus maximus

Hamstrings group

Gastrocnemius

Soleus

CONTRAINDICATIONS SPECIFIC TO BODY FARADIC TREATMENTS

In addition to the general contraindications and those for electrical treatments (see Chapter 3 Topic 1) specific contraindications for facial faradism treatments are:

- **loss of skin sensation (see Topic 4, tactile sensitivity test, which should be performed before treatment)**
- **muscular disorders**
- **highly nervous clients**
- **metal pins and plates**
- **high blood pressure**
- **nervous disorders**
- **migraine**
- **sinus**
- **any area of the body where severe discomfort is experienced during treatment**
- **sunburn**
- **pacemakers**
- **circulatory disorders**
- **muscle fatigue**
- **IUD (coil)**
- **first few days of menstruation.**

Note: The stimulation of the nerve endings will produce a sensation of tingling, which you should warn your clients about prior to increasing the current to achieve a contraction.

ELECTRODES USED FOR FARADIC TREATMENTS

There are several different types of electrode that can be used for faradic treatment:

- **an indifferent or passive electrode, dampened with saline solution and attached to the client, with an active disc electrode covered in lint or heavy gauze soaked in saline solution to increase conductivity**
- **a twin electrode containing both a passive and active electrode, moistened with a saline solution.**

FARADIC TREATMENTS
SUGGESTED PADDING LAYOUTS

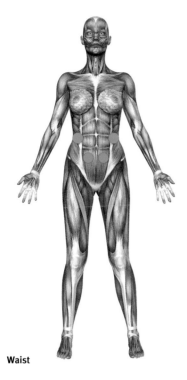

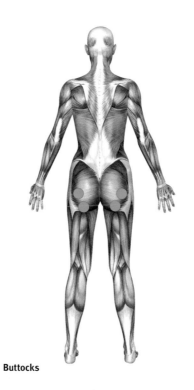

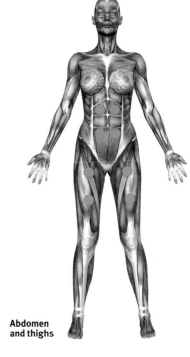

Waist

Buttocks

Abdomen and thighs

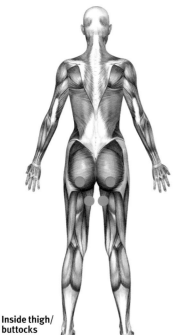

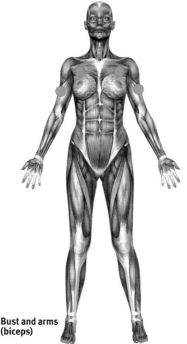

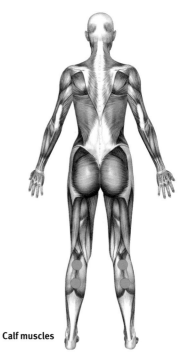

Inside thigh/ buttocks

Bust and arms (biceps)

Calf muscles

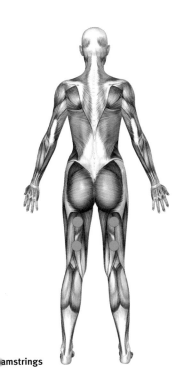

amstrings

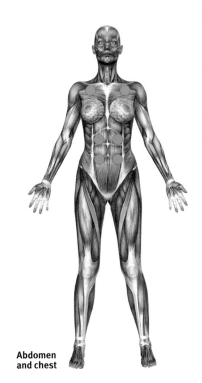

Abdomen and chest

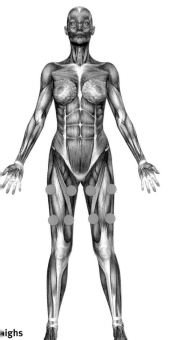

ighs

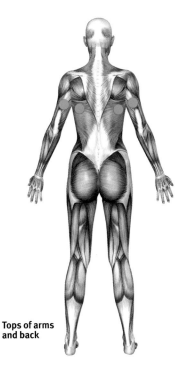

Tops of arms and back

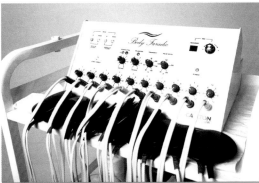

PREPARING FOR FARADIC TREATMENT

1. Discuss all aspects of the treatment with your client, including the tingling sensation mentioned above prior to full contraction of the muscles.
2. Carry out a tactile sensitivity test.
3. Check all plugs, wires and attachments. Ensure they are not loose or trailing.
4. Check all the electrical equipment you will be using on yourself first.
5. Make sure your client is comfortable.
6. Cleanse the client's skin with antiseptic in the area where the pads will be placed. Ensure all cream and/or oil is removed from the skin's surface.
7. Make sure you are in a position to see and adjust the controls easily.
8. Always follow the manufacturer's instructions for the machine you are using for any faradic treatment, as these can vary considerably.

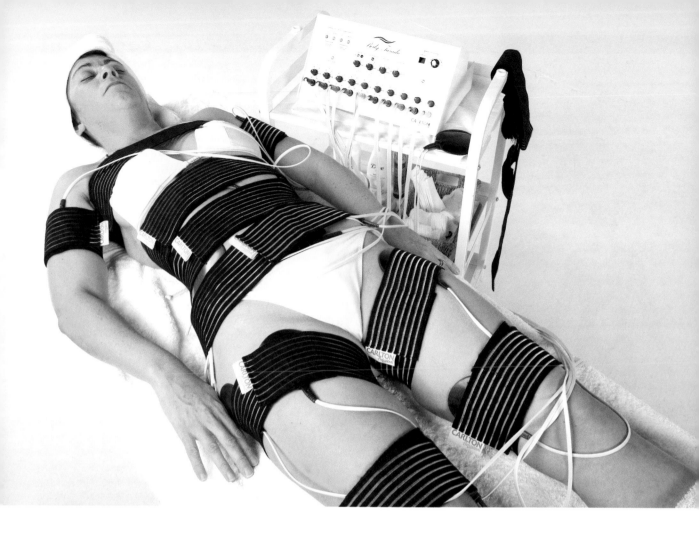

CARRYING OUT FARADIC TREATMENT

1. Test the machine on yourself first by holding a faradic pad on the top and bottom of your hand ensuring you can feel the current. Zero the frequency dial. Turn the machine off and re-sterilise the pad.

2. Wipe over the faradic pads with antiseptic. Position the faradic straps on the client first. Soak cotton wool in saline solution (1% dilution of salt in water) then wipe over the faradic pad before placing on the skin. This improves conductivity and muscle point response and reduces skin irritation.

3. Start placing the faradic pads on the side of the client furthest away from you ensuring you thread the wires through the bottom belt.

4. Repeat until all relevant pads are placed on either the belly or the motor point of the muscles to be exercised. The more accurately the electrode is placed, the stronger the contraction.

5. Check all the frequency dials are on zero then turn the machine on.

6. Turn up the intensity of the current ONLY when the electrode is in the stimulation period, NOT during the interval.

7. Increase the intensity until the client feels a prickling sensation. Then increase slightly more until a full contraction is seen. Move onto the next set of pads and bring them up to contraction working your way through all the areas to be treated.

8. Once all the muscles are contracting re-check the first set to ensure they are still fully contracting as they may get used to the current and need a little more stimulation in which case the intensity should be increased.

9. Leave the muscles to passively exercise for between 15 up to 40 minutes depending upon the general fitness and muscle tone of the client.

10. Do not leave the client alone and ensure that the machine is well away from them so that they cannot turn up the dials themselves.

11. Turn the current down before moving the electrode or repositioning pads.

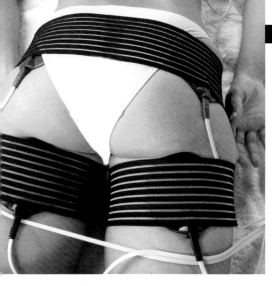

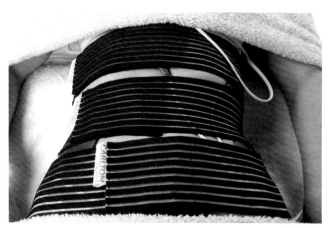

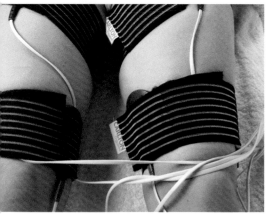

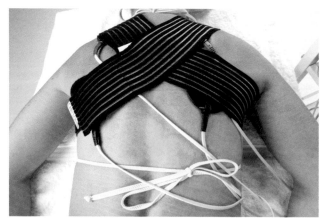

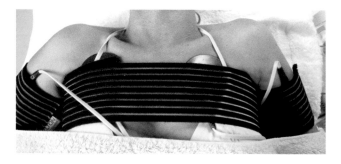

12. At the end of the treatment during the stimulation interval turn the machine off centrally, then immediately turn all intensity dials to zero.
13. First remove all the faradic pads from the client in reverse order to the sequence in which they were applied. This ensures wires do not tangle and equipment can be re-used with minimum of fuss. Sterilise the faradic pads as you remove them.
14. Remove the straps and neatly fold them up on the trolley in size order.
15. Wipe over the areas of the client that were treated.

AFTER FARADIC TREATMENT

1. Remove any remaining saline from the client's body with damp cotton wool. Apply powder to dry the area.
2. Continue with any further treatment.
3. Update client records after electrical to carry out a faradic treatment.

Endpoints
By the end of this topic, you should understand:

- the effects of faradic treatments
- contraindications to faradic treatments
- how to prepare for a faradic treatment.

TOPIC 6: MICROCURRENT TREATMENTS

Originating as a sports physiotherapy and Bell's palsy treatment, Microcurrent Electrical Neurotransmuscular Stimulation (MENS) has been successfully adapted to use its toning and firming effect as a cosmetic treatment to rejuvenate and recontour facial muscles. It is also used on the body to lift and treat muscles. It works by using a very low frequency microcurrent to stimulate the golgi tendon organ, which helps protect muscles and keeps them toned and active. Microcurrent treatment is gentle and relaxing and suitable for all ages and skins. Treatment time is up to one hour, with a routine of several treatments a week for several weeks recommended, then moving to a less frequent maintenance programme.

EFFECTS OF MICROCURRENT TREATMENTS

Microcurrent treatments are used to:

- **improve muscle tone by tightening and firming dropped contours, refining body lines, enhancing and defining muscle tone**
- **increase blood and lymph circulation and metabolism, removing toxins and waste and bringing nourishment to the skin**
- **improving skin tone and colour**
- **increase cellular regeneration.**

CONTRAINDICATIONS SPECIFIC TO MICROCURRENT TREATMENTS

In addition to the general contraindications and those for electrical treatments (see Chapter 3 Topic 1), specific contraindications for microcurrent treatments are:

- **loss of skin sensation (see Topic 4, tactile sensitivity test, which should be performed before treatment)**
- **muscular disorders, such as muscular sclerosis**
- **metal pins and plates**
- **excessive dental**
- **pacemakers**
- **heart conditions**
- **diabetes**
- **varicose veins**
- **dysfunction of the nervous system**
- **pustular acne**
- **when muscle relaxants have been prescribed.**
- **muscle fatigue**
- **IUD (coil)**
- **first few days of menstruation pace maker body piercing.**

PREPARING FOR MICROCURRENT TREATMENTS

1. Check the client's record card. Discuss all aspects of the treatment with your client, including the tingling sensation mentioned above prior to full contraction of the muscles
2. Carry out a tactile sensitivity test.
3. Check all plugs, wires and attachments. Ensure they are not loose or trailing.
4. Check all the electrical equipment you will be using on yourself first.
5. Make sure your client is comfortable.
6. Cleanse the client's skin with antiseptic in the area where the pads will be placed. Ensure all cream and/or oil is removed from the skin's surface.
7. Make sure you are in a position to see and adjust the controls easily.
8. Always follow the manufacturer's instructions for the machine you are using for any microcurrent treatment, as these can vary considerably.

ELECTRODES USED FOR MICROCURRENT TREATMENTS

There are several different types of electrodes that can be used for microcurrent treatment. They may be either microcurrent electrode pads, probes (single or dual), gloves, hands (as in indirect high frequency treatment), or a combination.

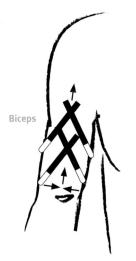

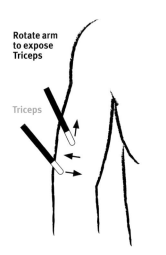

Rotate arm
to expose
Triceps

Biceps

Triceps

Biceps
With arm relaxed, palm facing forward,
place electrode flat either side of muscle,
apply pressure, lift and hold for 5 seconds.
Working from the elbow to the shoulder,
apply 5-6 lifts.
Repeat 4-5 times.

Triceps
With arm relaxed and turned in (palm of
hand on couch) or across clients chest apply
the same movements as for Biceps (8).

With hand on hip offering resistance thereby creating a natural contraction, repeat
moves 6 and 7, but with a flat electrode, not tip.

Remove excess gel and complete treatment by massaging the area with an appropriate
medium for 2-3 minutes.

Repeat procedure on the other arm.

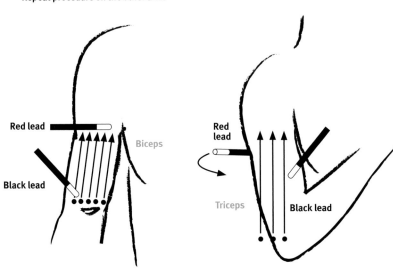

Red lead

Biceps

Black lead

Red
lead

Triceps

Black lead

Biceps
With arm relaxed, palm facing forward,
place one electrode (red lead) flat edge, on
deltoid muscle just above armpit and hold
stationary. With the tip of the other electrode (black lead) move towards stationary
electrode – medium pressure,
rapid movement.
Work from elbow to shoulder.
(approx: 10 strokes repeat 6 times).

Triceps
With arm rplaced across client chest, place
one electrode (red lead) flat edge, on top of
deltoid muscle and hold stationary.
With the tip of the other electrode (black
lead) repeat movement as for biceps (6).

CARRYING OUT MICROCURRENT TREATMENTS
Safety
Always follow the instructions appropriate to
the machine you are using for any microcurrent
treatment, as these may vary considerably.

1. Apply an electrolytic gel to the client's skin to
   improve conductivity and reduce skin irritation.
2. Select the waveform, frequency and current
   according to the client's skin condition. Unlike
   faradic treatments, microcurrent causes little
   or no visible contraction of the muscles, and
   so, for their comfort, you must be sensitive to
   the client's responses to the current.
3. Use dual probes or pads to stimulate specific
   muscles and produce a lifting effect moving
   the larger toward the smaller in a smooth, even
   motion ensuring you cover the whole area.

AFTER MICROCURRENT TREATMENTS
1. Remove any remaining gel with damp
   cotton wool.
2. Wipe the electrodes with a sanitiser and place
   in a sanitising cabinet.
3. Continue with any further treatment.
4. Remember to provide appropriate after-care
   advice – for example a good skin care routine
5. Be sure to update client records after electrical
   treatments. Sell your client a course of
   treatments in order to optimise the benefits of
   the micro-current treatment.

Endpoints
By the end of this topic, you should understand:

- the effects of microcurrent treatments
- contraindications to microcurrent treatments
- how to prepare for a microcurrent treatment
- how to carry out a microcurrent treatment.

TOPIC 7:
VACUUM SUCTION

Vacuum suction is used to stimulate lymphatic drainage and the vacuum massage movements also increase venous and lymphatic circulation. It is beneficial for inch loss and drainage of toxins especially conditions like cellulite.

The first treatment should be carried out with careful checking of the skin's reaction. If successful the treatment can be repeated, preferably about three times a week in a ten-treatment course, increasing the length of treatment time for maximum effect.

GENERAL EFFECTS OF VACUUM SUCTION

Vacuum suction treatment is used to:

- improve elimination and absorption of waste products through the lymphatic system
- improve skin texture through desquamation
- nourish skin and improve skin colour by stimulating circulation
- maintain skin firmness.

CONTRAINDICATIONS SPECIFIC TO VACUUM SUCTION TREATMENT

In addition to the general contraindications and those for electrical treatments (see Chapter 3 Topic 1), specific contraindications for vacuum suction treatments are:

- broken capillaries/thread veins
- fine, sensitive, loose, crepey skin
- bruised or broken skin
- bony areas
- loss of skin sensation (see Topic 4, tactile sensitivity test, which should be performed before treatment).

THE APPLICATOR/CUP

The applicator is a perspex/ glass cup, attached to an electrically driven vacuum pump, which creates a partial vacuum when placed on the skin. Cups come in varying shapes and sizes to suit different parts of the body or different functions. The amount of negative pressure used to create the vacuum is varied to suit the condition and flaccidity of the skin. There should be no more than 20% lift in the tissues as bruising or capillary damage could occur.

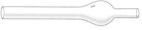

Pore blockage
Used to remove specific areas of blockages which group together and need intensified treatment i.e chin area. Also used for anti-wrinkle treatment.

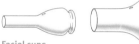

Facial cups
There are two sizes of facial cup ventouses. Used for lymph drainage massage or general cleansing, lifting and toning treatments.

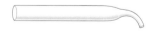

Comedone
The small round opening is placed over the comedone, ensuring that the pressure is exerted evenly on the surrounding tissue.

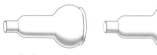

Body cups
Two sizes available for body work. The size of the cup selected will depend on the amount of fatty tissue in the area being treated.

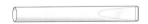

Lymph drainage
The flat head ventouse can be used for most vacuum therapy treatments, it will cleanse the pores whilst ensuring that the skin is not over pressurised. It can also be used ti work in the facial lines or give a lymph drainage massage.

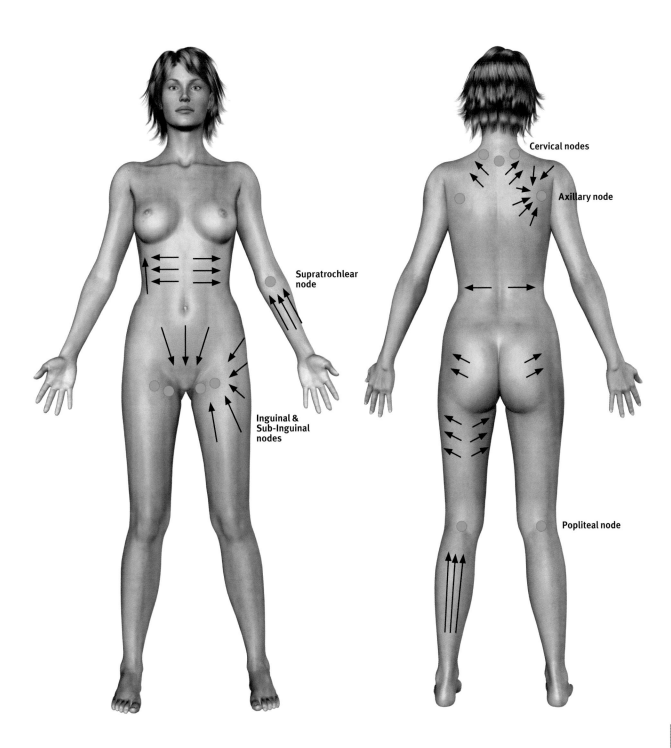

Supratrochlear node

Inguinal & Sub-Inguinal nodes

Cervical nodes

Axillary node

Popliteal node

Body vacuum therapy

PREPARING FOR VACUUM SUCTION TREATMENT

1. Discuss all aspects of the treatment with your client.
2. Check all plugs, wires and attachments. Ensure they are not loose or trailing.
3. Check all the electrical equipment you will be using on yourself first.
4. Make sure your client is comfortable.
5. Lightly spread some oil over the area to be treated.
6. Make sure you are in a position to see and adjust the controls easily.
7. Always follow the manufacturer's instructions for the machine you are using for any vacuum suction treatment, as these can vary considerably.

THE GLIDING METHOD

1. Place the cup on the skin of the area to be treated and turn on the machine. Adjust the vacuum to a suitable level for the area to be treated.
2. Slightly lift and use gliding strokes towards the nearest lymph nodes.
3. Break the suction of the cup by placing your finger close to the rim of the cup and gently depressing the skin to release suction. Then repeat the stroke between three to ten times on the same strip of tissue before moving on half the width of the cup repeating the process until the whole area has been covered.

Safety

4. Never pull the cup directly off the skin as you may create bruising and or broken capillaries. Always ensure that the suction has been released first. Each strip of tissue should be treated three to six times prior to moving on by the width of half a cup.
5. Follow the pattern of strokes indicated in the diagram, working towards the lymph nodes.
6. Observe your client's skin reaction, checking that your client remains comfortable throughout the treatment.

AFTER VACUUM SUCTION TREATMENT

1. Use damp cotton wool or sponges to remove any remaining product from your client's skin.
2. Continue with any further treatment if vacuum suction is part of a larger treatment.
3. Detach, clean and thoroughly cleanse all tubing in detergent and place it in a sanitised container. Detach and clean the cups in detergent first, then place in a sanitising cabinet.
4. Be sure to update client records, as after any electrical treatment.
5. Sell the client a course of treatment to ensure maximum benefit.

Endpoints

By the end of this topic, you should understand:

- the general effects of vacuum treatments
- contraindications to vacuum treatment
- how to prepare for vacuum treatments
- how to perform vacuum treatments.

TOPIC 8:
INFRARED TREATMENTS

Infrared rays work by penetrating the superficial epidermis, producing heat, warming and soothing the body tissues. In addition to their therapeutic effects on the skin, infrared treatments generally help people to relax and give them a feeling of wellbeing.

INFRARED TREATMENTS

Infrared rays work by penetrating the superficial epidermis, producing heat, warming and soothing the body tissues. In addition to their therapeutic effects on the skin, infrared treatments generally help people to relax and give them a feeling of wellbeing. The heat lamp is especially beneficial for clients with aching muscles and areas of tension. Infra-red treatment is also often used as a preparatory treatment before massage.

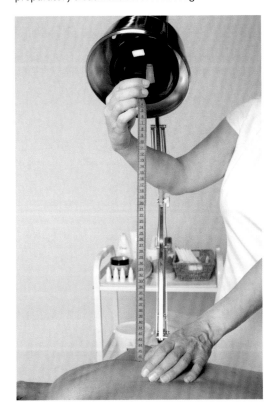

GENERAL EFFECTS OF INFRA-RED TREATMENTS

Infrared treatments are used to:
- **increase circulation including increased activity of sweat glands**
- **heat the blood and warm the tissues, creating erythema prior to deeper treatment such as massage**
- **dilate the pores**
- **relax tense muscles**
- **preheat tissues prior to further treatment**
- **increase absorption of products**

CONTRAINDICATIONS SPECIFIC TO INFRARED TREATMENTS

In addition to the general contraindications and those for electrical treatments (see Chapter 3 Topic 1), specific contraindications for infra-red treatments are:
- **loss of skin sensation (see Topic 4, thermal sensitivity test, which should be carried out before treatment)**
- **hypersensitive skin**
- **diabetes**
- **sunburn**
- **pacemaker**
- **body piercing.**

SAFETY PRECAUTIONS SPECIFIC TO HEAT LAMP TREATMENT

Using a heat lamp creates more potential hazards in the salon. Following a checklist can help ensure that your client enjoys the treatment safely.

CHECKLIST
Advantages to false tanning

1. Check the lamp, ensuring that:
- there are no trailing, loose or frayed wires
- there are no dents in the canopy of the lamp – this would cause the tissues to be heated unevenly creating 'hot spots'
- the lamp has been warmed up away from the client (the lamp should be switched on at least ten to fifteen minutes before it is needed to reach its maximum intensity)
- the lamp is positioned over the tripod leg and not directly above the client
- the lamp has been tightened to prevent any movement once it is in position
- the lamp should be placed a minimum of 50 cm away from the most highest point on the area to be treated (and usually not further than 1m). For a reminder of the inverse square law, see opposite
- you are following the manufacturer's instruction about use, distance and angle of the lamp
- the lamp is clean, dust free and in good working order
- the lamp is positioned safely away from the client in order to cool down.
2. Check that:
- your client has removed contact lenses and all jewellery before treatment
- your client's skin is suitable for infrared treatment (see thermal sensitivity test and contraindications on page 204)
3. Check your client's skin reaction throughout treatment.
4. Never leave your client alone during treatment.
5. Do not use the lamp for longer than the specified time.

SAFETY AND THE INVERSE SQUARE LAW

The intensity of rays varies inversely with the square of the distance from the lamp. Thus, the intensity of radiation at 30cm is four times that at 60cm and eleven times that at 1m, so 1 minute at 30cm distance is the equivalent of four minutes at 60cm and eleven minutes at 1m.

Because of this you must always adhere to manufacturer's instructions on exposure time and distance of the lamp from the client's skin.

Endpoints
By the end of this topic, you should understand:

- the general effects of infrared treatment
- contraindications to infrared treatment
- safety precautions for infrared treatment
- the implications of the inverse square law for safe infrared treatment.

TOPIC 9:
GALVANISM AND IONTOPHORESIS

Galvanism is an electrical treatment that passes a direct current through the skin. It can be used on all skin types, and its particular effects depend on the polarity used:

- A positively charged active electrode with a positively charged gel or a negatively charged active electrode with a negatively charged gel, causes the active ingredients to be absorbed into the skin (iontophoresis). Generally iontophoresis (or ionisation) passes substances into the skin to break down fatty deposits and cellulite. It works for several hours after the treatment finishes. These treatments work on the principle that opposite poles attract, while like poles repel each other.

EFFECTS OF IONTOPHORESIS

The general benefits that a client is likely to notice after iontophoresis are:

- acidic reaction on the skin
- moisturises and hydrates by introducing active substances deeper into the skin than is normally possible without the use of galvanic current
- firms and tightens the skin, breaks down fatty deposits and cellulite
- increases circulation – taking waste products away from the area refines the texture of the skin on the body.

GENERAL EFFECTS OF THE GALVANIC CURRENT

The general benefits that a client is likely to notice after galvanic treatment are:

- stimulation through increased circulation
- break down of fatty deposits by introducing the relevant substances in to the body tissue deeper then would be possible without the galvanic current.

SAFETY PRECAUTIONS FOR GALVANIC TREATMENTS

- Check contraindications.
- Check the machine is in good working order and has no loose wires or cracked plugs.
- Check the machine is placed on a safe surface, e.g. a professional trolley.
- Check there is no water on the trolley.
- Prepare the skin appropriately, including tactile sensitivity test.
- Check the machine on yourself first by using the facial electrodes on yourself (forearm) to check the current is flowing.
- Talk to the client throughout the treatment and ensure you inform them of the effects of the treatment.

SPECIFIC CONTRAINDICATIONS

Specific contraindications for galvanic treatments are:

- sinusitis
- loss of skin sensation (see Topic 4, tactile sensitivity test, which should be carried out before treatment)
- braces, large number of metal fillings or metal pins or plates in the face/head.
- pacemaker
- IUD (coil)
- body piercing.

PREPARING FOR GALVANIC TREATMENTS

- Discuss the treatment beforehand with your client:
- check for contraindications
- explain the sequence of the treatment
- describe to the client the sensations that they may experience, (e.g. a slight tingling in the skin.)

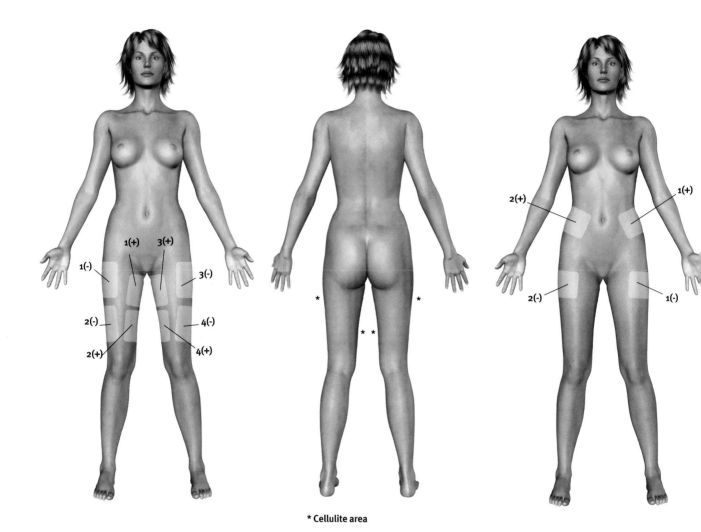

1(+)
3(+)
1(-)
3(-)
2(-)
4(-)
2(+)
4(+)

2(+)
1(+)
2(-)
1(-)

* *

* *

* Cellulite area

ask your client to tell you if they experience these sensations. You can use this information together with careful visual observation to judge duration and intensity of treatment and the point at which to turn the current down. In the case of galvanism, providing the client can feel the 'prickle' of the current you can be assured that the machine is working and the current is flowing – therefore there is no reason to increase the intensity any further. This usually happens at a maximum of 1–2 amperes.

Explain that if they feel uncomfortable, they should tell you and you will then reduce the amperage (intensity) or stop the treatment. The treatment should cause only gentle skin stimulation.

1. Carry out a tactile sensitivity test.
2. Check all plugs, wires and attachments. Ensure they are not loose or trailing.
3. Check all the electrical equipment you will be using on yourself first.
4. Make sure your client is comfortable.
5. Cleanse the client's skin with antiseptic in the area where the pads will be placed and ensure all cream and/or oil is removed from the skin's surface.
6. Make sure you are in a position to see and adjust the controls easily.
7. Always follow the manufacturer's instructions for the machine you are using for any galvanic treatment, as these can vary considerably.
8. Apply the necessary gel (see below).

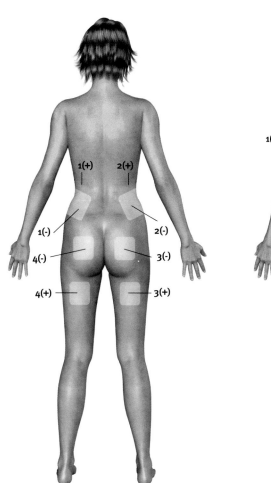

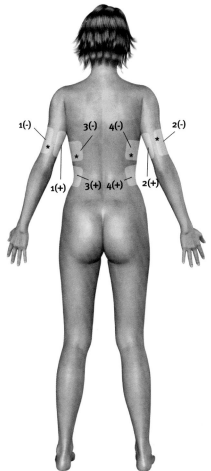

* Cellulite area

THE ELECTRODES

The body electrodes consist of metal plates attached by wires or graphite pads directly to the galvanic machine. They come in pairs one of which is positive and the other is negative.

Polarity can be switched depending upon the type of machine and the type of product used therefore always check manufacturer's instructions. Galvanism works on the principle that opposites attract thereby drawing substances deeper into the body tissues than is normally possible.

THE IONTOPHORESIS (IONISATION) TREATMENT

1. Soak the galvanic sponges in water to ensure they are damp.
2. Apply galvanic gel to the main area to be treated with a sanitised brush.
3. Apply straps close to the area to be treated ready to hold the galvanic electrode and sponges in place.
4. Encase the metal galvanic plates within the soaked sponges. If any metal touches the skin it could cause a galvanic burn.
5. Place a separate single damp piece of sponge over the area to be treated underneath the straps, and then place the galvanic plate on

top of it. Place the indifferent electrode on the opposite side to draw the ionised substance towards it.

6. Turn the current up slowly according to the amount of resistance in different parts of the body. For instance, lower the intensity of the current when working on the bony areas. The client should feel a slight prickling sensation which is sufficient to indicate that the current is flowing taking the active substance deep into the skin. Build the treatment up from a minimum of ten minutes to a maximum of twenty

7. Turn the current down slowly at the end of the Treatment then immediately switch the machine off. Slide the electrodes from underneath the straps in the reverse to how they were placed on the body. Wash the sponges immediately and wipe down the electrodes with sanitiser. Wipe over the area of the body treated with warm soapy water and the area where the indifferent electrode was placed to remove all galvanic substances. Be very careful to remove from the indifferent side as caustic soda may build up and could cause a caustic burn if left on the skin.

CONCLUDING THE GALVANIC TREATMENT

1. Detach all electrodes and sanitise and store them appropriately. Suggest some exercise the client can perform in between treatments.
2. Sell the client a course of treatment.
3. Be sure to update client records after electrical treatments.
4. Give the client suitable skin and home care advice.

Endpoints

By the end of this topic, you should understand:

■ the effects of iontophoresis
■ safety precautions for galvanic treatments
■ how to prepare for and perform galvanic body treatments.

TOPIC 10:
MECHANICAL MASSAGE

Vibratory massage is a method by which the client can be massaged by mechanical means. It can take several forms, and is especially suitable for remodelling of excessive adipose areas although it does not substitute weight loss.

Gyratory vibrator

The Gyratory vibrator machine delivers mechanical massage by means of a number of different shaped heads which are applied to different parts of the body by the therapist. In essence the technique follows manual massage (see Chapter 9: Massage techniques) in that it replicates the different strokes and movements, depending on which head is used.

Training is required to understand both the fundamental principles of massage, and how to deliver vibratory massage using the Gyratory massage machine.

The Gyratory massage machine

This machine can be free-standing and is a heavy piece of equipment which is generally regarded as specialist. Newer models are smaller and can be easily rolled around on castors to access different parts of the client's body.

Benefits of Gyratory massage

There are many benefits to Gyratory massage, for both the client and the therapist. Generally this equipment can perform far deeper massage than manual methods, as well as better penetration into fatty areas of the body, breaking down adipose tissue and helping to contour the body. Whilst this is often a reason why therapists team Gyratory massage with weight loss programmes, it should

• DID YOU KNOW?

The Gyratory massage machine was originally designed in the 1950s by a French welder by the name of Henri Cuinier. Working for Renault, Cuinier saw the chance to adapt the machinery he used to weld cars to help his polio stricken wife recover faster using massage. He developed the machine which quickly became world renowned for its quality.

be stressed that this method of massage is not a replacement for diet and exercise. Although it can be a very appropriate supplement to these practices.

Advantages:

Deeper massage than manual means, meaning more pressure can be used for the client so long as they are comfortable with this less personal manner of treatment, making it preferable for clients who might otherwise be self-conscious about massage.

Electronic delivery means this is a far less intense technique for the therapist to apply, allowing longer treatments.

Different applicator heads

The Gyratory massage machine uses many different applicator heads which can vary with equipment. Generally, however, they fall into three categories:

Sponge heads. These can be flat or curved in shape depending on the area to be massaged. Generally massages begin with a round flat sponge head, and a curved sponge is used to mould to legs and arms. They replicate the effleurage stroke in massage.

Hard rubber heads. Rubber heads mimic petrissage strokes and can perform a variety of functions.

Those with pin shaped rubber protrusions can slough away rough skin and stimulate blood-flow, whilst 'football' and 'egg box' shaped domed heads can provide deep penetration to areas of heavy adipose or thick tissue and muscles which mimic petrissage movement.

Spiky and brush heads are used to stimulate the lymphatic system and deliver a light percussion style stroke.

Effects of Gyratory massage

- Lymphatic circulation
- Provides blood circulation
- Sloughs away dead skin
- Relaxes muscles and eases muscle pain
- Penetrates deeper than manual massage making it particularly suited to treat cellulite and dispersing fatty tissue.

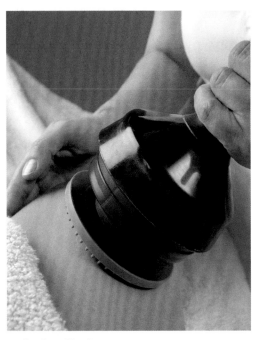

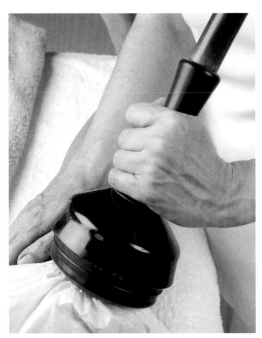

A spiky shaped head

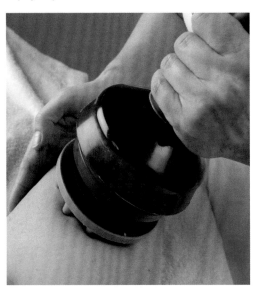

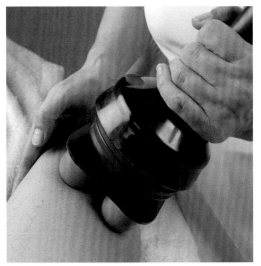

'Egg box' shaped domed heads

Method of application

1. Cleanse the area to be treated and check for contraindications.
2. Apply powder to add slip to the area to be treated.
3. Select the appropriate head to begin with which would normally be effleurage.
4. Select the applicator head to be used and ensure it is securely fitted.
5. Switch the machine on away from the client then check the machine on yourself first.
6. Apply the head to the area to be treated gradually increasing the pressure as the treatment progresses
7. Use long sweeping strokes towards the heart and the nearest lymph nodes either leading or following with your free hand to maintain contact throughout the treatment with your client.
8. Once the whole area has been successfully covered change the applicator head to petrissage and apply it in small circular motions taking care to feed the tissue into the applicator. Do not press down on to the bone as it could be uncomfortable for the client.
9. Once the whole area has been covered change to the percussion head which is spiky in appearance and helps to vigorously stimulate the circulation and aid with desquamation.
10. Once the whole area has been covered and an erythema is present in the tissues, massage the area again with the effleurage head to finish off.
11. Repeat on all appropriate areas of the body avoiding any boney areas.
12. When the treatment is complete wipe over all the massage heads with sterilising solution and store them in a sterilisation cabinet.

After care

1. Remove any excess powder from the area.
2. Advise the client on appropriate diet and exercises to supplement the vibratory massage treatment.
3. Continue with any further spa treatments.

Contraindictations to Gyratory massage

Please refer to page 155 of the massage techniques chapter for a full list of the contraindictations to Gyratory massage.

Endpoints

By the end of this topic, you should understand:

- Gyratory massage, gyratory massage applications and equipment
- advantages of Gyratory massage
- audio sonic massage and applications.

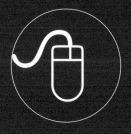

DON'T FORGET
TO LOGIN TO GAIN ACCESS TO YOUR **FREE** MULTI-MEDIA LEARNING RESOURCES

- ☐ **Over 40 minutes of instructional videos of all the key treatments**
- ☐ **Lesson plans and multiple choice and essay questions**
- ☐ **Interactive games and quizzes to help you to test your knowledge**

To login to use these resources visit
www.emspublishing.co.uk/spa and follow the onscreen instructions.

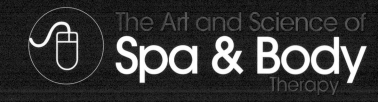

The Art and Science of
Spa & Body
Therapy

Index

Index continued

Index continued

Index continued

Index continued

Index continued

Index continued

Index continued

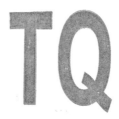

Index continued